Close to the Sun

THE JOURNEY OF
A PIONEER
HEART SURGEON

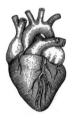

STUART JAMIESON

RosettaBooks®
New York, 2019

The patients named here were identified in the news media at the time, together with their progress. Those who were not identified publicly are referred to only by first names, which have been changed, as have their physical characteristics. Names and physical characteristics have also been changed by others who are identified only by their first names.

To my daughters,
Alexandra and Victoria.

"I warn you to travel in the middle course, Icarus,
if too low the waves may weigh down
your wings, if you fly too high the fires will scorch
your wings. Stay between both."

—Ovid

RosettaBooks®

CONTENTS

FOREWORD

One of the most significant scientific advances of the past century is the ability to perform surgery on the human heart. Cardiac surgery ranks in importance with space travel, computers, antibiotics, control of communicable diseases, and other major breakthroughs made during the twentieth century.

In his memoir, Dr. Stuart Jamieson presents a vivid account of his experiences as a member of the so-called second generation of cardiothoracic surgical pioneers. In a highly engaging and readable manner, he describes the background and formative influences that led him to choose a surgical career. Like many other creative individuals, he had a fascinating early life that did not necessarily prepare him for his later professional accomplishments. Of particular interest are the stories he tells about the adventures he experienced during his developmental years in southern Africa.

Dr. Jamieson's surgical career was marked by a new, aggressive approach to the treatment of cardiopulmonary disease. Because of his interest in heart and lung transplantation, he helped introduce many technical modifications in these procedures. He also helped pioneer strategies for overcoming tissue rejection, which had previously impeded favorable long-term outcomes. One of the most important breakthroughs to which he contributed was the early use of the immunosuppressant drug cyclosporin, which substantially improved the results of transplant procedures. Perhaps the most significant of his many accomplishments, however, is the operative procedure he devised to solve the difficult problem of pulmonary embolism. That operation is among the most challenging and complex of all cardiopulmonary procedures. His results with it are unequaled.

This book includes intimate insights into the lives of pioneers in heart surgery and transplantation, weaving the history of heart and lung surgery into Dr. Jamieson's own history. With its generous illustrations and human interest stories about both patients and physicians, *Close to the Sun* should appeal to medical professionals and the general public alike. Complex medical situations have been made easily understandable to laypersons.

On a personal note, I recall being asked many years ago by the British Heart Association to give an invited lecture at the Brompton Hospital. Arriving at Heathrow Airport, I was met by a bright young surgeon who introduced himself as Stuart Jamieson. He was then a registrar at the Brompton Hospital and had been assigned to escort me during my visit. We enjoyed the first of many enjoyable conversations. I was impressed by him at the time, and that excellent impression has continued over the years. I am proud of our friendship.

Denton A. Cooley, MD
Founder and president emeritus
Texas Heart Institute
Houston, Texas

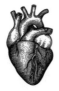

PART ONE
AFRICA

CHAPTER ONE
STARTING OVER

The plane from Cape Town was crowded. Most of the passengers were white and appeared well-off, dressed in crisp khaki and headed home from shopping in South Africa for the essentials they could no longer find in Zimbabwe. I'd heard that in the years since the civil war had toppled white rule in the country formerly known as Rhodesia, it had become nearly impossible to buy anything that wasn't made there. Now a trip to the store for toothpaste required international travel. We flew over dusty plains and bouldered outcroppings. As the plane traveled into Zimbabwe and made its descent, I saw that the airport at Bulawayo, which I remembered as a grand place, was little more than a crumbling airstrip in the middle of a scrubby field. We landed, pulled up to the terminal, and got off at Gate 5—an amusing conceit, as it was the only gate. Inside I noticed a few game heads on the walls, forlorn reminders of a different time.

The lines in the immigration area were long and slow. The thump of papers and passports being stamped echoed monotonously. When I at last reached the front, I handed my passport to a young black officer in a starched uniform. He looked at it for a long moment and then up at me.

"You were born here, in Bulawayo?" he asked.

"Yes," I answered.

"Welcome back, sir," he said, stamping my passport and waving the next in line forward.

I rented a car and drove through town, which took only a few minutes. After thirty years, everything looked familiar but in disrepair. The streets were crowded with people. AIDS had begun its hollowing out of the population, and nearly everyone I saw was either young or old. There was nobody in between, and nobody seemed to have anything to do. A little beyond the edge of town opposite the airport, I came to our old house. It looked more or less as it had, though it was now surrounded by a high wall. A steel gate guarded the entrance to the driveway. A sign of different times. As I looked the place over, two young boys tore around the property on small motorbikes. I remembered how my father often spent his weekends perched on a low stool weeding the lawn, looking smart in his bush hat and listening to the cricket matches on a transistor radio. Presently, a Mercedes swept up to the gate. An impatient-looking white woman honked the horn, and a gardener ran over to let her in before going back to his watering.

I headed for Whitestone, the boarding school I had gone off to as a young boy. The dirt road was now tarred, and houses stood in rows on either side where the bush had once crowded in. There were children in the schoolyard, both black and white. This I'd expected, though the fact that half were girls brought me up short. Whitestone had been a boys' school in the grim English tradition when I'd attended, run by incompetent instructors whose ignorance and cruelty were thought to be the best sort of influence on the leaders of the future. This

14

had been a torture then reserved for whites only. I'd hated every minute of it. The students no longer wore khaki but were now smartly turned out in crimson jackets with a bird embroidered on the front pocket. The school itself appeared little changed. I ruefully contemplated the motto over the door: *Veritas Omnia Vincit.* Truth conquers all. It's a concept that's easy to believe until you've lived long enough to see through it.

Farther out of town, I stopped in at Falcon College, where I attended high school, "college" being an English term for secondary school. Falcon was located on the site of an abandoned gold mine, whose plain stone buildings had been converted to classrooms and dormitories. I remembered the swelter of classes beneath those corrugated iron roofs as the African sun burned its way across the day. Now there was air-conditioning. And just as at Whitestone, the school was fully integrated. Students went about campus in mixed groups, seemingly oblivious to race. They proved a point I would not make out until years later, when a classmate wrote about it in the Falcon newsletter. Falcon had become a color-blind oasis in the heart of Africa, a living model for what some had once hoped all of Rhodesia could become. That was not to be.

My father was a doctor. He had sided with the liberals in Rhodesia. They favored an orderly transition away from white minority rule. The exclusion of blacks from the colonial government was wrong, he believed, and would end either well or badly. White rule did end, though not while my father was alive to see it, and not in the way he hoped it would. Rhodesia became Zimbabwe in a cataclysm of bloodshed and terror. Its black citizens, most of them uneducated and possessing no knowledge of the outside world, were ill prepared for liberal, Western-style democracy. The concept of "one man, one vote" is fair enough. But when the average person cannot read or write, does not know that the oceans and continents exist, has no idea even that there are other countries, other people—then the idea of self-rule falls down, because a vote is going to be for sale. And they were. Zimbabwe is a country now run by a corrupt, authoritarian black government that exploits its citizens more brutally than the white government ever did. That is Zimbabwe's history and its torment.

I'd come back to Africa to see all this for myself, but also because I'd recently experienced a calamity of my own. I'm a heart surgeon. My career had taken off in the pioneering days of heart transplantation, a life-saving operation that I'd helped make routine. At a young age, I'd been given my own cardiac center at a major university in America and turned it into the world's busiest heart-transplant hospital. And then, abruptly and unjustly, I was forced out, my reputation in tatters. I'd been a success in every way except at perceiving the envy that gnawed at the people I worked with. I loved what I was doing and assumed that everyone around me did, too. I was wrong.

One of my favorite stories when I was growing up was the Greek myth of Daedalus and his son, Icarus, who escaped their confinement on the island of Crete by flying away on wings Daedalus fashioned from branches of willow bound with wax. Daedalus, fearful of the hazards of the journey and seeing his son's rapture at the prospect of flight, warned Icarus to fly safely above the sea, but not so near the sun as to melt his wings. Icarus ignored this advice to stay on the middle course, instead soaring high into the sky. And when his wings melted, he fell into the sea and was lost.

The lesson of Icarus is that excessive pride or self-confidence can be fatal, though I never saw it exactly that way. To me Icarus was not foolish, but bold. Wanting to do something great isn't hubris, to my way of thinking, but neither is it entirely safe. Extraordinary achievement does not lie along the middle course. Heart surgery is not for the timid, and in the beginning every breakthrough carried immense risk. Doctors and their patients flew not just close to the sun but directly at it. For me it was intoxicating. True enough, when I did fall, it was a long way down. I'd lost almost everything. But soon I'd be ready to go up again. My visit to Africa was a prelude to starting over.

I have always enjoyed heights, the thrill of pioneering achievement, despite the risks.

CHAPTER TWO
BULAWAYO

My story begins in a place and in a way of life that no longer exist. In a sense, I am homeless, cut off from the world I knew growing up in the heat and dust and stark beauty of southern Africa. And yet that Africa lives in my memory. Since I have left, I have traveled to all parts of the world and operated on paupers, presidents, and princes. But in the cold still of the dawn, wherever I am, my mind falls quickly back to those early mornings on the Zambezi River. In whatever country in the world I find myself, a part of me is still there.

I reminisce over the early cool dawns on the river. The mist lay still on the water and crept along the riverbank. Cape buffalo browsed in the bush, hulking black shadows that moved noiselessly among the trees, pausing now and then to stare balefully in my direction as they chewed. They breathed clouds of steam in the morning light. There was a peace then that I never since have achieved.

I remember, too, our summer home, a cottage called Serondella, on the Chobe River, a tributary of the Zambezi. I learned to water ski on the Chobe, a perilous enterprise on account of the crocodiles and hippos with which we shared the river. And I remember our home, Raigmore, in the town of Bulawayo, Southern Rhodesia, where I was born in 1947. My parents named the house for the place in Scotland where they met during the war. It was a sprawling one-story home, painted white, with many windows and an encircling veranda that looked out over several acres that were ours. The windows had bars on them for security—everyone's did—though I don't remember ever feeling this was necessary. The house had no air-conditioning and a fireplace that was unneeded except for a few weeks in the cooler months. There was a guesthouse in the back, and behind that were the servants' quarters. My father had a large study that was lined with books and maps on which he marked the routes of many of Africa's pioneering explorers. In the evenings after dinner, he would sit in his study alone with his pipe and read about the history of Southern and Central Africa. He seemed to know everything about the part of Africa that we called home.

My mother delivered me at the Lady Rodwell Hospital, which stands to this day, sun splashed in crisp, colonial white-wash with a red slate roof, though I doubt that it is still strictly a maternity hospital, and certainly it is no longer exclusively for whites. Surrounded by palm trees and a neatly kept lawn, Lady Rodwell was adjacent to Bulawayo General Hospital, one of the hospitals at which my father worked and where he later died. There was no hospital then for blacks.

We moved to Raigmore, in a suburb of Bulawayo called Hillside, when I was still a young child. I had an older brother, Chris, who'd been born in England, and eventually a younger sister named Margy. My earliest memories are of the gardens at Raigmore. The large lawns were lush during the rainy season from November to February, the Rhodesian summer. The rain came in thunderstorms, torrents that lasted a few hours, after which the sun reappeared and the air was clear and fresh. Jacaranda trees lined the flower gardens, which contained flame lilies, orchids, and hibiscus. In the winter months, the rain ceased. Sometimes the grass withered from lack of watering, but it always recovered when the rainy season returned.

My favorite tree was a marula in the lower garden in the front of the house. Although there were no elephants in Bulawayo—the only wild animals routinely encountered there were snakes—everyone in that part of Africa knew that elephants love to eat the fruit of the marula tree. In late summer, when the fruit has fallen to the ground and turned a soft yellow, elephants have been known to eat so much that the fruit ferments in their stomachs and they get drunk. Elephants can be dangerous, and tend to be more so when inebriated, but it is a great sight to see an elephant barely able to stand, or see one careening drunkenly through a grove of trees, shearing off branches as it goes. Many years have gone by since I enjoyed a marula, but the bittersweet taste is still fresh on my tongue.

Like many of the white families in Bulawayo, we had a swimming pool. There was also a tennis court. It was seldom used but was an object of fascination for me, as it required the constant attention of our gardeners. The court had an earthen surface, not clay, but dirt from giant anthills that was saturated with used engine oil and then pressed flat with a huge roller made of steel and concrete. It took two gardeners to pull it, and it was a mystery as to how the unwieldy contraption had come to be kept within the walls and wire netting surrounding the court. The only answer had to be that it was there first. Despite the continuous labor invested in maintaining the court, in truth its greasy, uneven surface was never satisfactory for the tennis. We weren't much interested in playing, anyway, in the heat and sun, and eventually it was paved over.

I did use the tennis court for another purpose, however. I learned to shoot on it. There was a solid stone wall at one end that was an ideal backstop for target practice with a pellet gun my father bought for us. I must have been six or seven. I discovered that I had a talent for shooting. I could hit anything with that gun, even dragonflies as they flew around the swimming pool. Being a good shot was important in Africa. One day it would save my life.

....

Bulawayo sits on a plain, in the southwestern quadrant of what was then Southern Rhodesia, between the equator to the north and the Tropic of Capricorn to the south. It is some four thousand feet above sea level, with a moderate climate that is never cold and rarely sweltering. It is a young city, a town, really, that was barely fifty years old when I was born. Its history before then was bloody, and began when it was first colonized not by white Europeans, but by an invading force of black Africans coming north out of South Africa, which was then known as the Cape Colony.

These were Zulu people, led by a great field general named Mzilikazi. Mzilikazi had been a military leader under the legendary king Shaka Zulu. But after a rift with the king in 1823, Mzilikazi led a contingent loyal to him north, across the Limpopo River, into what would later become Southern Rhodesia, and then Rhodesia, and in the current chapter of this history, the country we now call Zimbabwe. Mzilikazi and his band wandered for a number of years, conquering local clans wherever they were encountered, killing freely and burning villages to the ground. Once, when Mzilikazi got separated from his forces and was presumed dead, one of his sons took charge. When Mzilikazi unexpectedly returned, he immediately executed the son and all who had supported him.

Eventually Mzilikazi settled his people in a rugged region called the Matopos Hills, where they became known as the Matabele, and the area under their control Matabeleland. The Matabele remained warlike, measuring their wealth in the livestock they owned and the number of enemies they had killed. The displaced tribe, a group called the AmaShona, fled to the north. The conflict between these two groups continues to this day; Robert Mugabe, the longtime president of Zimbabwe and a member of the Shona tribe, is responsible for many atrocities against the Matabele.

Mzilikazi died in 1869. Kuruman, the son of his senior wife, disappeared mysteriously. Lobengula, another son by a lesser wife—Mzilikazi had two hundred wives—seized control, killing those who opposed him. It was to be a brutal reign, maintained through regular executions of anyone suspected of disloyalty. Sometimes the charge was witchcraft, though no excuse was needed. Lobengula settled himself in a cluster of huts surrounded by a stockade—a *kraal*—to the north of the Matopos Hills that came to be known as *Gu-Bulawayo*, "The Place of Slaughter." This would one day become my home.

Toward the end of the 1800s, white ivory hunters crossed over the Limpopo River and into Lobengula's land. They included the famous explorer and elephant hunter Frederick Courteney Selous. In 1888, a contingent representing Cecil Rhodes, the soon-to-be prime minister of the Cape Colony and head of the British South Africa Company, arrived at Lobengula's *kraal* looking to negotiate a monopoly on gold and other mineral deposits. The talks stalled, as other white adventurers—Dutch Boers and the Portuguese—tried to convince Lobengula he was being swindled. As tensions escalated, it seemed that Lobengula might shortly resolve the impasse by simply killing every white man he could find.

At the eleventh hour, a Scottish physician named Leander Starr Jameson arrived on the scene. Jameson was named after an American tourist, Leander Starr, who had saved Jameson's father from drowning. Because of poor health, Jameson had gone to South Africa in 1878 and started a medical practice at Kimberley, where he treated many influential people. He also became a close friend and confidant of Cecil Rhodes. Jameson traveled to *Gu-Bulawayo* at Rhodes's behest and calmed the situation there by treating Lobengula for gout and an eye condition. Lobengula was so delighted that he made Jameson an *inDuna*—an adviser and ambassador. Jameson was the only white man to have undergone the initiation ceremonies for this honor.

Jameson concluded a deal with Lobengula granting exclusive mining rights to the British in exchange for money and guns. It was stipulated that Lobengula would remain the ruler of his land, and anyone coming into it to dig would have to acknowledge his authority. The agreement was signed on October 3, 1888—the starting date for British colonization of Matabeleland.

Lobengula soon regretted his concession to the British and threatened war against the white colonists. There was animosity on both sides. Even the elephant hunter Selous, who had been Lobengula's friend and supporter, was disillusioned by the Matabele. On a visit to England in 1889, Selous was invited to a breakfast by the Anti-Slavery Society in honor of two Matabele envoys. Selous declined, explaining in a letter, "It does strike me as incomprehensible that your Society above all others should have chosen to so honor the envoys of a tribe such as the Matabele...a people who, year after year, send out their armies of pitiless, bloodthirsty savages and slaughter men, women and children indiscriminately—except for those just the ages to be slaves..." Selous was referring to the Matabele's treatment of the Shona.

On September 12, 1890, a military volunteer force of settlers, organized by Cecil Rhodes and guided by Selous, founded Fort Salisbury, named after Lord Salisbury, the British prime minister at the time. Located about 250 miles northeast of Bulawayo, Fort Salisbury subsequently became known simply as Salisbury, the colonial capital. It is now called Harare.

In 1893, Leander Starr Jameson, by then the administrator for Rhodes's British South Africa Company, ordered the Matabele's armed regiments out of the area of *Gu-Bulawayo*. This was a direct challenge to Lobengula, and war became inevitable. Since the whites were badly outnumbered, Jameson decided he should strike the first blow. Troops were gathered in Salisbury and in neighboring Bechuanaland, now Botswana. A third column was raised at Fort Victoria, under the command of an officer named Allan Wilson.

The three forces met at *Gu-Bulawayo*, but Lobengula had vanished. Dr. Jameson ordered a pursuit, and on December 3, 1893, colonial soldiers reached the banks of the Shangani River, 120 miles north of *Gu-Bulawayo*, at sunset. Captain Wilson took twelve men to reconnoiter the far bank, intending to return before dark. But when Wilson discovered Lobengula's camp, a gathering of seven thousand armed Matabele, he sent back a message saying that he would remain on the far side of the river for the night and attack at first light to capture Lobengula. Twenty men were sent across to reinforce Wilson's scouting party.

The next morning the thirty-two-man Wilson patrol found itself surrounded by thousands of Matabele. Wilson summoned three men to cross back over the river for help. One was Frederick Burnham, an American from Minnesota, who had come to Africa looking for more adventure after fighting in the Indian wars. He was joined by Pearl Ingram, known as Pete, another American, and William Gooding, an Australian. Burnham, an experienced scout, told Wilson that he thought reaching the other side was impossible, but that he and his two companions would try. Fighting their way through the Matabele, then swimming the flood-swollen Shangani River, they discovered the main force fighting for its life against a Matabele ambush. There would be no more reinforcements coming.

The Wilson patrol ringed their horses around themselves and shot them to provide a protective barricade. A fierce battle was waged until their ammunition ran out. Every man was wounded. Wilson was among the last to die. Later, the Matabele warriors told the story of Wilson's valor. The badly wounded men had loaded their rifles and passed them to Wilson, who continued to fire. When the ammunition was spent, the men of the patrol who could stand rose and sang "God Save the Queen." Wounded in both arms, Wilson, staggering and without a weapon, advanced toward the Matabele. Though one of the Matabele stabbed him, Wilson continued his approach. The warrior shouted, "This man is bewitched; he cannot be killed!" and threw away his spear. Wilson then fell forward on his face, dead. The Wilson patrol had been outnumbered by more than two hundred to one.

Allan Wilson's "last stand" was one of the Rhodesian origin stories that I learned and revered as a boy. Though my parents had come from other places, I never thought of myself as anything but Rhodesian. To me, men like Selous and Jameson, Wilson, and Rhodes were heroes—founding fathers as noble and courageous as the founders of the United States, where I have lived for many years and of which I am now a citizen. Like this country's founders, Rhodesia's were men of their time, brave and far-sighted, but also perhaps imperfect and dependent on a class system based on race that was fraught with inequality and was ultimately unsustainable. The bones of Allan Wilson and his men were buried at the Matopos Hills, at a place Rhodes named World's View. Rhodes was buried there in 1902, and later his friend Leander Starr Jameson was placed in a grave beside him. A monument to Wilson and his men stands there today, unmolested despite the current strife in the country.

Lobengula died two months after the destruction of the Wilson party, knowing that the inexorable advance of the white men could not be resisted forever. Before his death he compared himself and his kingdom to a fly that had been eaten by a chameleon: "The chameleon gets behind the fly, remains motionless for some time, then he advances very slowly and gently, first putting forward one leg and then another. At last, when well within reach, he darts his tongue, and the fly disappears. England is the chameleon, and I am that fly."

Although Lobengula was gone, the Matabele army had not been defeated. In March 1896, there was open rebellion once more. With first the Matabele, then the Shona three months later, the tribes erupted in violence, slaughtering hundreds of white settlers—a shocking 10 percent of the European population. The Second Matabele War, as it is now known, is celebrated in present-day Zimbabwe as its First War of Independence.

During the Second Matabele War, the *Gu-Bulawayo* morphed into Bulawayo. It was besieged by the Matabele forces, and a defensive encampment was established there. The situation was grim—each evening nearly a thousand women and children slept on the ground within an inner defensive wall of wagons. Rather than wait for attack, the settlers mounted patrols, called the Bulawayo Field Force. Their leaders included Selous and also Frederick Burnham, one of the Wilson patrol's three survivors. These quick-strike parties patrolled the countryside, rescuing settlers as they could. Although outnumbered, they soon attacked the Matabele directly. Twenty men of the Bulawayo Field Force were killed and another fifty wounded within the first week of fighting.

Relief forces arrived in late May 1896 to break the siege. An estimated fifty thousand Matabele retreated to their stronghold in the Matopos Hills south of Bulawayo. The turning point came when Burnham and a young scout named Bonar Armstrong made their way through to the Matopos Hills looking for the spiritual leader of the Matabele, Mlimo, who claimed to be invulnerable to the white man's bullets. Burnham and Armstrong tethered their horses near the mouth of a cave where Mlimo lived, a sacred place to the Matabele. When Mlimo returned, he started his dance of invincibility with the Matabele looking on in awe from outside. Burnham shot Mlimo through the chest. He and Armstrong then fled on horseback just ahead of a thousand stunned Matabele warriors in pursuit. The two men outran their pursuers all the way back to safety at Bulawayo.

That autumn, Cecil Rhodes, accompanied by Burnham, went unarmed into the Matabele camp in the Matopos Hills and persuaded the warriors to lay down their arms, ending the Second Matabele War in October 1896. Within a year white colonists had successfully settled in much of the territory known as Southern Rhodesia. In 1953 Southern Rhodesia joined with Northern Rhodesia, across the Zambezi River to the north, and with Nyasaland, to form the Federation of Rhodesia and Nyasaland. The Federation lasted ten years, until Nyasaland broke away and became Malawi and Northern Rhodesia became Zambia. Alone again, Southern Rhodesia became just Rhodesia in 1965. That same year, in an attempt to quell a rising call for integration of the government, Rhodesian prime minister Ian Smith issued the Unilateral Declaration of Independence from the United Kingdom. This would lead to years of unrest and ultimately civil war.

Frederick Selous had been wounded during the siege of Bulawayo. Afterward, he returned to his ranch not far from

Bulawayo and rebuilt his house at Essexvale, which had been burned by the Matabele, who also stole all of his cattle. The house, where Selous watched elephants from his veranda, was situated on a bend in the Lunga River, near where I went to school. My stepfather later owned this ranch. The epic saga of imperialism and conquest that was Rhodesia mingled in me with a deep love of that place and its native people. Friends today say, usually with suspicion, that I am a colonial.

But how could I not be?

....

And so I was born in wild Africa, in Bulawayo, less than a lifespan after the Second Matabele War. The Matopos was one of my favorite haunts. I loved to visit the cave where Frederick Burnham shot Mlimo, where I lived with ghosts past, and where the history of Rhodesia felt alive to me. The cemetery at Rhodes's World View stood atop a granite hill. I climbed there often, to sit among the graves and the Wilson memorial, and to look out over the valleys below. We used to pick the small "resurrection plants" from between the rocks. To all appearances the plants were brittle and dead. When taken home and put in water, they turned green again.

This was my heritage, the story of my country. The places from which my family had come were abstractions to me— remote and alien. My English grandfather had emigrated to Australia in 1893, where he taught chemistry at Scotch College in Melbourne and authored several widely used science textbooks. Grandpa, a tall, elegant figure, always wore a three-piece suit with a hat. He carried a walking stick or rolled-up umbrella at all times, regardless of the weather. He smoked, always using a cigarette holder, and carried his cigarettes in a silver case. I only met him once. He came to stay with us for six months during the African winter, from March until

August 1952, when I was five. I remember him as mysterious and aloof.

My father, George Arthur Jamieson, was born on Palm Sunday, March 23, 1902, in Gawler, South Australia. I don't know much about his early life, though it was apparently colorful. He became a doctor, earned enough to invest in racing horses and gold mines, and was on one occasion thrown out of Raffles, the famous Singapore hotel, for being drunk and disorderly. Later in life he was reserved. I don't think I ever heard him raise his voice. He was thin, just over six feet tall, and had a mustache. He wore a suit and waistcoat most of the time, and smoked Old Navy cigarettes. Strangely, he sounded English. Apparently his father would not permit him to speak in an Australian accent.

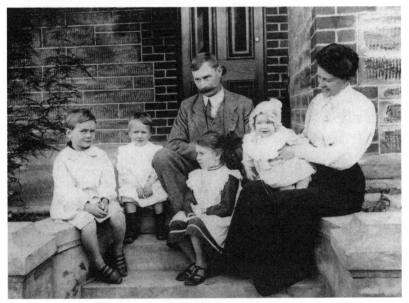

My grandfather and grandmother in 1908.
My father is on the left.

During the Second World War, by then a middle-aged bachelor, he went to Britain and joined the Royal Air Force, rising to the rank of wing commander. His primary duties were medical, but he also flew missions over France. Posted in Scotland, he became aware of a young woman who worked on the base as a plotter in the fighter operations room, moving small placards around on a map with a long stick to track the locations of planes aloft. Janet Winifred Pascall was eighteen, twenty years younger than my father. She was almost six feet tall, pretty and sure of herself. And she was used to the attentions of the men on the base. One day my father came up to her and announced that he owned a yacht and planned to go sailing later that day. If she cared to join him, he said, she should be at the dock at three in the afternoon. She was.

They married in 1945.

My parents told me little about the war, but my mother once mentioned the distress she experienced at hearing over the radio the screams of pilots shot down in their burning planes. She had been drinking and laughing with many of them the previous night in the pub. After the end of the war, my father's adventurous nature took over. They moved to Southern Rhodesia, where he set up practice as an ophthalmologist and ear, nose, and throat doctor. My mother and my brother, who was then a small baby, came out in late 1946 on a troop ship under appalling conditions. When she arrived at the docks in Cape Town, all of their luggage had been lost. They were delayed a few days before embarking on the three-day train trip through southern Africa to Bulawayo. My mother received a warm welcome from my father at the train station in Bulawayo. I was born eight months and two weeks later.

My mother's parents eventually came to live with us at Raigmore. I remember their first visit when I must have been a few years old. They flew out from London in a civilized fashion, before jet aircraft were in commercial use. They came in a flying boat that landed on a series of large rivers as it progressed southward. They would anchor at nightfall and dine and sleep on the plane. I suppose they must have landed on the Nile, and the Congo, and the great lakes of Africa. Their final water landing was on the Zambezi River above the Victoria Falls at Livingstone. They then took another airplane to Bulawayo.

For several weeks my parents had been telling me that I was finally to meet Granny and Grandpa. I was excited, even though I was not sure who Granny and Grandpa were. Since there was no municipal airport at Bulawayo, commercial planes landed at the military airbase, where my father, who had served in the RAF reserve, was always welcome. After I met my grandparents at the airport, I continued to ask, "Yes, but where are Granny and Grandpa?" The concept of extended family was new to me, because we lived so far away. During this trip, my mother's parents decided to move to Africa to live with us.

I am not sure my father was entirely happy about this, but he built them a house seventy-five yards from ours. My grand-father became my great friend and confidant. When I was con-fined to bed for three months with brucellosis at about the age of ten, he used to play draughts (checkers) with me. I got to know him well during that time. Grandpa liked to play bowls at the Bulawayo bowling club. Twice a week he would come out of the cottage wearing a green striped blazer and white trousers, with special bowling shoes. He carried his bowls in a little case, inscribed "WWP." These were his initials, Walter Wilfred Pascall, but he said it stood for "World's Worst Player." That couldn't have been true, because he represented South-ern Rhodesia in the Empire Games in Australia.

Life at Raigmore had a comfortable colonial rhythm and formality that I found agreeable. Our parents did not coddle us in any way. On the contrary, they were physically remote from us, loving but not demonstrative about it. The children were to be seen and not heard, and were certainly not allowed to be an inconvenience. We dressed for dinner every evening without exception, my father in black tie and Chris and I in jackets and ties. The meal was attended by our houseboy, Simon, who was of course black and I thought handsome in his starched white uniform and red fez. We had a nanny, Emily, a soft, round Matabele woman, who wore a blue dress with a starched white apron and white cap. I loved the smell of her skin, always scented with the Palmolive soap she used. She had trouble pronouncing *Palmolive* and called the soap *"Plumleaf insopi," insopi* being Zulu for soap, a European invention. When we sat outside on the sunny afternoons, I would trace patterns and do drawings on her skin with a twig. I loved Emily and spent a lot more time with her than my parents. We would sing the English nursery rhyme "Who Killed Cock Robin" in Zulu. I spoke Zulu better than I spoke English until I went off to boarding school. Emily was part of the family and lived in a house at the back of the garden.

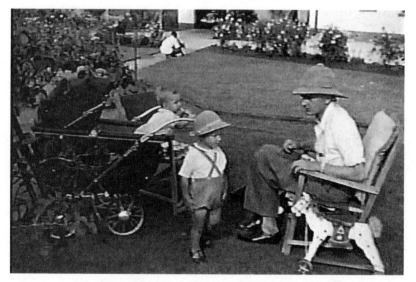

At Raigmore with my father and brother, 1948.

We had other servants at home besides Emily and Simon. We had a cook and several "garden boys," who looked after the grounds, wearing khaki shirts untucked over their khaki shorts. Barefoot, unlike the house servants, they were usually seen with a wheelbarrow or garden hose. It was a happy household, one that to my young mind comported perfectly with the world and everyone's station in it.

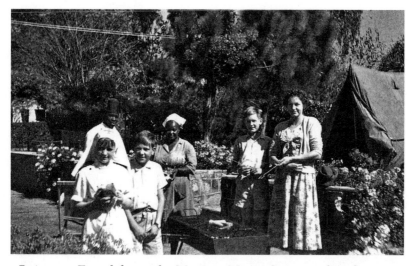

Raigmore. From left to right: My sister Margy, Simon (in his white uniform and fez), me, Emily, my brother Chris, and my mother.

Bulawayo was still a dusty provincial town with broad streets designed by Cecil Rhodes to allow a wagon behind a full span of sixteen oxen to do a U-turn. The streets were so wide that cars could park nose-in on either side, and then in two rows nose to nose down the middle, still leaving two lanes of traffic going each way. There were only three traffic signals in town. Bulawayo had some industry—a cement factory and a slaughterhouse. The white population was about five thousand, while there were around 250,000 blacks. Most blacks who didn't work and stay at white homes lived in small cement houses in a part of town known as "the location." Only whites paid taxes, and so it was a struggle to find the money for the education and infrastructure that would make black advancement possible.

Cecil Rhodes, who died three days after my father was born, was a towering figure in this isolated place. Bulawayo in most ways was still an outpost not unlike the old pioneering towns of the American West. Rhodes had made his fortune in the diamond fields of Kimberley by buying up the small diamond operations. He was financed in this by the Rothschild bank. He died at forty-eight, leaving a provision in his will for the famous Rhodes Scholarships at Oxford University. Rhodesia was named after him, a legacy now gone.

I remember a curious thing, a project my father undertook that continued for several years. We had a long, unpaved driveway that entered the property from a dirt road. There were pillars on either side of the entrance, but no gate. The drive curved up toward the house and circled back on itself. One day, my father decided to pave the driveway with bricks. These were not cobblestone pavers, but actual bricks, the sort you might build a wall with, turned on their sides and laboriously set in place in a zigzag pattern, three at time, first this way and then the other. He started at the house and worked toward the road. The driveway had to be excavated and leveled by hand to bring the bricks flush with the ground, and then meticulously prepared with sand, on top of which the bricks were carefully tapped in place.

My father did all this work by himself. Every Sunday he'd sit on a small canvas stool, setting bricks. Progress was made by the inch, season after season, and after several years we began to wonder if the work would ever be finished. And then my father abruptly halted when the brick surface was still some twenty feet short of the road. It was strange. I don't think he wanted to finish. It was if he thought his life might be over if he did.

There was a social scene in Bulawayo, and my parents enjoyed it. They liked their friends and they liked their whiskies at the end of the day. A small difficulty was that my father also liked to invite black guests to the garden parties we held at our house from time to time. This was considered improper, and it also caused problems with our servants, who felt they should not be compelled to wait on other blacks, as this was beneath their dignity. My father would patiently explain that they worked for him and that meant taking care of any guests he decided to entertain. Simon and the others complied, but I don't think they were happy about it.

When I was about eight years old, my father was instrumental in the construction of an African hospital in Bulawayo called Mpilo, where blacks could finally receive medical attention. He usually worked there a couple of days a week. He never charged his patients at Mpilo, but I think he found it rewarding in other ways. Blacks in Africa often developed cataracts, and my father changed many lives with the surgery that corrects this problem. Mpilo is an African word for "life." Today, Mpilo Central is the largest hospital in Bulawayo and the second largest in all of Zimbabwe, and there is a plaque in the corridor to my father's memory.

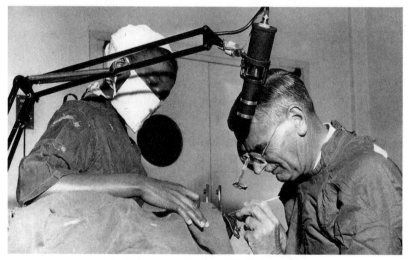

My father operating at Mpilo Hospital.

Given the brutal history of *apartheid* in neighboring South Africa, it's natural to think that the racial divide in Rhodesia was the same. But this was not the case. To be sure, there was a sharp demarcation between the races. Whites were the ruling class, and blacks were the servants. So the blacks were exploited, no question. And they were also denied self-governance. The government was white. But neither whites or blacks regarded one another with malice. There was not the kind of resentment between the races that existed in South Africa, or even in America, for that matter. Everyone was treated with respect. No one was forced to work, and certainly nobody was owned as they once were in this country. It's hard to explain, but the racial environment felt nontoxic when I was growing up. And that undoubtedly helped to mask the underlying injustice of the situation, the unspoken but abiding tensions that would one day explode.

From my earliest memories, I knew I wanted to be a doctor. I was inspired by the dedication of my father, and by the thought of making a difference in people's lives. And I thought that surgeons made the biggest difference. I loved the idea that a surgeon could fix people. At a young age, I would "operate" on grapes, removing the pits and sewing the skin up again with a needle and thread. But medicine was far in my future, and looming ahead was boarding school, a break with childhood from which you never returned. Being sent away to a good school was considered a privilege, an expensive one. I remember how it started.

I was left standing at the end of a long driveway in the hot afternoon sun, with a tin trunk by my side. A black beetle stirred in the sand at my feet as my parents drove away in the dust. I stared up at my new home, Whitestone School. It was only on the outskirts of Bulawayo, but it might as well have been in another country. I had left home for good. I was eight years old.

CHAPTER THREE
WHITESTONE

Whitestone was a school for 120 sons of gentlemen. The school's name was a translation of a Matabele word *Matcheumslope*, meaning "white stone," which was the name of the river that ran down through the *kopjes* into reservoirs behind the dams below the school boundaries. *Kopje* is an Afrikaner term for an isolated hill or rocky outcropping.

Students at Whitestone were between six and thirteen years old and were divided into six grades, or "standards," as they were called in Rhodesia. Though I went home for the holidays, from then on being at home was only temporary. I had become a visitor at Raigmore. Whenever it was time to go back to Whitestone after a break, I got a simple wave from my parents before they turned away.

I held it together for a few days. I missed my mother terribly. It had not occurred to me that she would no longer be a part of my daily life. And I missed a sense of ownership over my own space, with my own things safely in it. At eight years old I was not ready for this, not ready to be on my own. Our dormitory was on the second floor at the top of a stone stairway. It was a long, high-ceilinged room with wooden floors and rows of beds on either side—like a hospital ward—with mosquito nets that were drawn up to the wall at the head of the bed each morning. I lay awake on my straw mattress that first night, and for many nights after, with my face pressed to the pillowcase because my mother had touched it when she packed my trunk. I had been allowed one blanket from home, and I held on to it, trembling, listening to the sounds of boys I didn't know breathing close by in the echoey void.

The matron in charge of our dormitory was Miss Byerly. She was called, but not to her face, "Ma" Byerly. A large Afrikans woman, she wore starched white clothes with heavy, white lace-up shoes, and a nurse's cap perched on her straight black hair. She was a burly person, and intimidating. I am not sure what qualified Miss Byerly to be a keeper of boys. Perhaps none was required. Nobody challenged her authority.

Miss Byerly strode through the dorm with a *sjambok*, a five-foot-long whip made of stiff rhino hide that she rarely put down. One night I was awakened by a noise that sounded like a pistol shot. Miss Byerly was standing at the doorway with her *sjambok* in her hand, which she had whacked across the doorway. The lights went on. All the boys sat up in bed, wide-eyed with terror. Miss Byerly walked down the line of beds, lashing the wooden floor with the *sjambok*. She said that she had heard somebody talking, which was forbidden after lights out. She demanded to know who it was.

Silence.

Miss Byerly squared her shoulders and said calmly that she was prepared to thrash every boy within an inch of his life if the culprit did not "own up" to his crime. Finally, a small, angelic blond boy, with pale blue eyes and curly hair, fell out of his bed sobbing. He knelt on the floor in front of Miss Byerly and admitted he had been talking, just a word or two.

"Mercy, Miss Byerly," he pleaded, "mercy."

Miss Byerly studied the boy for a moment. Then she tore off his pajama shirt, stepped back, and struck him sharply with the *sjambok*. A welt rose on his back. Again the whip fell with a loud crack. And again. When the welts began to bleed, Miss Byerly stepped back and let the whip down at her side. Then she turned on her heel and walked out, snapping off the lights as she went. No one made a sound. I'd never seen anyone beaten like that. It would not be the last time I did.

In the daytime we all wore khaki shorts with a short-sleeved khaki shirt. In the evenings the dress was khaki shorts with a khaki shirt and school tie. On winter evenings we wore a gray jersey with the neck in the school colors, red and green. Nobody ever needed a coat. White shirt, tie, and blazer were required for Sunday evenings, the only time we put on long trousers, even in the middle of winter.

We were sent home for our holidays just three times a year. These were momentous occasions for most of other students, who came from places like Salisbury, or who lived on farms in the outlying country, or were from the copper mining or farming areas of Northern Rhodesia or Nyasaland. For me the holidays were a bittersweet reminder of the distance between the life I had always known and the one into which I'd been thrust. Our house was probably only ten miles from the school, but in every way that mattered I was no closer to home than anyone else.

The separation from my family and the grim, prison-like atmosphere of Whitestone had a profound and permanent effect on me. I felt betrayed, abandoned. It didn't help that my brother, Chris, who was one year ahead of me, was also at Whitestone.

We'd grown up close, but now Chris was remote, and when he did speak to me it was usually to say something dismissive. I was the inconvenient and hopeless little brother. I didn't see how things could get worse. And then they did.

We rose at six each morning and went to our classrooms for homework before breakfast at seven. The school was chilly before the sun was fully up, and we shivered in our tropical khakis. We had to line up outside the classrooms for roll call in alphabetical order. When the J's were reached the call was "Jamieson major?" That was my brother. He responded "*Ad sum,*" I am here. Then it was "Jamieson minor?" "*Ad sum,*" I said, though I wished I wasn't. Waiting there for my name to be called in the cold dawn and knowing I would then have to respond in front of the whole school filled me with apprehension. It was as if a chasm had opened up between my brain and my mouth. Two words just five letters long—*ad sum*—threatened to choke me. Over the course of only a few days, each morning harder and more terrifying to me than the last, my heart racing and palms sweating even in the cold, I developed a stammer. Soon I had stopped speaking altogether except when absolutely required to do so. My humiliation only made the impediment worse. It would take me decades to get over that stutter. I have since given hundreds of speeches in my career and can speak comfortably before a thousand people. But even now there are words that I avoid because they remain difficult for me to say. Another lingering phobia is a meeting that begins with everyone going round and introducing themselves. I could spend an hour explaining a complex heart surgery, but the idea of speaking my own name fills me with dread. I usually say something about the weather instead, and if it goes well I risk "Dr. Jamieson" and hope to spit it out.

Breakfast was from seven to seven thirty. We made our beds after breakfast, before chapel and prayers. Shortly after I arrived at Whitestone, I found myself one day standing at the bottom of the stairway leading up to my brother's dormitory. Chris was nine, a year older than I. In the hierarchy of an English boarding school, a year's difference was like a generation. As a "new boy," I was not permitted to ascend the stairs to my brother's dormitory. So I had to wait for him so that we could walk together to chapel. I wanted to tell him how unhappy I was and how much I missed home. I needed to see my brother. As I waited for him, I started to cry. One by one, the older boys came down, ignoring me as they brushed past. Finally, one stopped and asked what was wrong. I said I wanted to see my brother. He went back up, and after a few minutes Chris appeared and rushed down the stairway. He didn't stop, but started off for the chapel. "Stop standing there blubbering like a baby," he said.

I felt even more alone.

Discipline at Whitestone was harsh and frequent. Beatings were common and were regarded as a natural hazard of daily life. One day, in the great hall where we had meals, an announcement was made that some students had been throwing soap at each other during the evening baths. This was to stop. I didn't pay much attention at the time.

Bathing was regimented at Whitestone. You were allowed exactly ten minutes. The water was to be four child's fingers deep, no more. Two boys bathed together, facing each other in the tub. To economize, the water was not changed between shifts. If your turn came toward the end, the bathwater was cold and had taken on a muddy appearance.

As it turned out, the rule breaker was me. The two baths in the junior dormitories were three feet apart. A boy called Jeffries in the other bath asked for the soap, which was always in short supply. Since it was a little too far to reach over, I lobbed it to him. An informant later told Miss Byerly that I had been throwing soap. This was an offense so serious that even a whipping on the spot with the *sjambok* would have been insufficient. I was reported to the headmaster. After being made to wait for several days in abject fear, I was summoned to the headmaster's office one morning after breakfast.

To get to the office, I had to walk down a long corridor and then descend a stair into the building occupied only by the teachers. No boy visited these halls unless they were to be subjected to severe discipline or informed of a family tragedy. The air of doom was oppressive. I was made to wait outside the master's study. The door finally opened, and I was ordered in. The headmaster was an Afrikaner named Van Heijst. His nickname was Frikkie, which was Rhodesian schoolboy slang for a condom. He was thickset and plodding and looked disgusted with me. A glass cabinet full of bamboo canes stood against one wall. One had been taken out and laid across the desk. The headmaster asked if I had anything to say for myself. I explained what had happened and that I had not really been throwing soap. "You boys," he said. "Always full of excuses. Bend over."

I reached for my toes while he lined up alongside me. For the worst offenses, you received six blows. "Six of the best," the saying went. No one ever got more, because after six lashes the flesh was raw and you didn't feel much anymore. My crime merited four. After a caning it was proper form to straighten up, shake the headmaster's hand, and say thank you. One could never cry.

On my return to the dormitory, all the others wanted to see the huge welts. The stripes would be visible as blisters and bruises two or three months later. A severe thrashing would leave your khakis bloody.

I learned two important things from my time at Whitestone. One was that life is not fair. The other was that physical pain is not a permanent injury.

....

Central Africa in the 1950s was mostly bush. The fringes of Bulawayo, where Whitestone was, were not particularly wild. There were hazards, including many varieties of venomous snakes, but dangerous large animals such as lions and leopards had been chased away and were now found twenty miles or more from town. The boys at Whitestone were all comfortable in the bush, and we knew how to look after ourselves. It was part of growing up in Africa. Whitestone only had one school rule. It was that you were to use common sense. My brother once fell out of a tree and broke his arm. As soon as his arm had been set and put in a cast, the headmaster beat him. The beating was not for climbing a tree, but for falling out of it.

The headmaster's numbers two and three were brothers, Douglas and Gerald Pennington. We called them DP and GP. DP had two canes he called *Swassa major* and *Swassa minor*. GP had a paddle that he called a butter pat that he used to keep order. It hurt just as much as a thrashing with the canes and kept everybody on his best behavior, but the brothers were decent people and fair with their beatings.

GP was a bachelor and never married. He taught Latin and mathematics. Gray haired, middle aged, thin, he walked with a slight stoop but was nevertheless an accomplished athlete and taught cricket and field hockey. DP was stockier, married, and had children. Among them was a son called Christopher, nick-named Kiffy. Kiffy was probably two years younger than me. Since he lived at Whitestone year-round and had the place to himself during the holidays, he was regarded as a kind of superior being. No one envied him his continuous presence at school, but it did give him the upper hand since this was his home as well as his school.

Kiffy had a talent for painting. There were bushman paintings in the caves and protected *kopjes* around Whitestone. Many thousands of years old, these Kaffir paintings, as they were called, depicted hunting scenes. We all knew where they were and visited them often to contemplate the wild humans who had made them so long ago. The Bushmen of times past had been small, no bigger than we were, and so many of the paintings could only be reached by a child capable of squeezing through small openings in the rock or by traversing narrow granite ledges. It was common to come across snakes in these cramped passages—usually cobras. If we didn't bother them, they generally just hissed and slithered away.

After a while, we began discovering new paintings. They were not in the same elegant and simple style of the bushman paintings we knew so well. Eventually, we discovered that Kiffy had created them during the school holidays. In time, Kiffy's counterfeits improved, though it was always possible to tell his from the originals. I sometimes wondered if they would somehow later be discovered and deemed an unusual school of prehistoric art.

On Sundays we were allowed out for the day. We could leave the school grounds but were to stay within prescribed areas. Going home was forbidden. We had to go in small groups and indicate a destination when we signed out. A group had to include at least three students, so that if one was injured another could remain with him while the third went for help.

I loved these outings and took every chance to go exploring. One of my favorite places was a large granite *kopje* a mile from school. It was a hard climb to get to the top, but when you did, you were rewarded with a view over a cluster of lakes called the Hillside Dams. There were caves there, too, with paintings on the walls and shards of old pottery lying about.

One of the most challenging climbs brought you to a rocky crest that was sheltered beneath a stand of trees where it was pleasant to sit. It was a favored haunt for small antelope and also rock hyraxes, which resembled large brown guinea pigs. We called them *dassies*. There was also evidence of wild goats, which we sometimes saw, though more often we came across their droppings. Once Chris went up there with me and we named the place Goat's Bog Island, "bog" being our slang for a latrine. I thought of it as a special place.

Although Rhodesia felt far removed from major world events, we knew that we lived in dangerous times, and that a nuclear holocaust could wipe out all life on earth. Chris and I swore a pact that no matter where we were, if the world ever turned completely upside down, we would meet at Goat's Bog Island. I found this a comforting idea. When I mentioned it to Chris many years later, he had no idea what I was talking about.

Rhodesia held dangers of its own. It was not unusual for a student, or a member of his family, to be killed by an animal or in some kind of accident. Fatalities increased dramatically during the civil war, and many boys with whom I went to school died in unhappy ways before they were twenty-five.

When I was nine, a classmate named McClaren was told to report to the headmaster. He was terrified and didn't want to leave the classroom. The teacher put her arm around his shoulder and led him out of the room down the endless corridor toward the headmaster's study. When she returned, the teacher closed the door and explained to the rest of us that McClaren's father had been eaten by a crocodile. We were to be kind to McClaren, as he would be upset.

We did our best to be sympathetic, though this was not a strong suit among young boys in boarding school. It wasn't long before the taunts began. How had McClaren's father been so careless as to have been eaten by a crocodile? McClaren took this hard at first but within a few days seemed back to normal.

I had my own close brushes with mortality. Once I fell off a wall onto my head, landing on some rocks about ten feet below. I was groggy and unsteady afterward. Since I was behaving strangely, I was taken to the sanitarium, our small school clinic that was run by a matron with little medical training. She was concerned enough to call my parents, and I was taken home. Waking up in my bed at home about eight that evening, I wandered around the house until I came to the drawing room where my parents were drinking whiskey with the neurosurgeon from town. They were discussing whether to open my skull to drain the blood that might have built up as a result of the concussion I had suffered. When I walked in, they looked relieved and helped themselves to another whiskey.

I had hepatitis at the age of ten. There were several cases of hepatitis at our school at the time. We were inoculated against various diseases at the beginning of term. Back then, the syringes and needles were reusable and not sterilized between use. Many boys were stuck with the same needle until it became too blunt to penetrate the skin. Whenever we saw a new needle being put on the syringe, there was a race to be first in line. Someone in the line ahead of me must have been infected, and I developed a desperate case of the disease. I was sent home when I became so yellow I was almost green. I was placed in my parents' bed, where I passed in and out of a coma as my mother stood at the bedside weeping. I think I nearly died.

Another close call was the time I was poisoned. Meals at Whitestone were rationed. There was never enough to eat. I was always hungry. And I found some of the food inedible, especially the burned black beans that were served to us every Friday evening. They always made me vomit. But we had to eat what was on our plates or face the consequences with Miss Byerly. I would eat a few mouthfuls, go outside to be sick, and come back again for a few more mouthfuls, until the plate was clean. Regurgitating those beans was better than the *sjambok*.

In November or December, when the rainy season replaced months of drought, flying ants would appear. They were actually termites. During homework sessions the lights in the classroom would attract flying ants by the thousands. Some would land on the floor. We would then catch and eat them. You pulled the wings off and chewed fast so that they didn't wiggle as they went down. They tasted like butter.

The dining room was also used as an auditorium and had a stage at one end. When I was in the fifth standard, about ten years old, we were rehearsing A *Midsummer Night's Dream*. I was Mustard Seed, one of the fairies. During rehearsals, I noticed some red crystals on the dining room table that looked like gelatin. They tasted awful. It turned out I had eaten fly poison. I ended up at the Bulawayo General Hospital. On recovering and returning to Whitestone, I was beaten for being so greedy as to eat from the table when it was not mealtime.

I never did play Mustard Seed, because shortly thereafter I contracted brucellosis and was once again confined to bed.

Brucellosis is an illness caused by drinking unsterilized milk or eating infected meat from animals. The first signs I had this disease were fevers and sharp pain in my left hip, especially at night. My hip joint was infected. I was sent home, and my left leg was put in traction. This was excruciating. I had twice-daily tetracycline injections. Sometimes I would cry out in the night in pain, which never abated. Either there was no pain medication or I was never given any. Though he must have been tired and faced a full day's work ahead, my father would hear me and come in to sit by my bed until dawn, when the pain became easier to bear. After three months of bed rest,

I was allowed to walk again, but only on crutches or using a "caliper," an instrument of torture disguised as a leg brace. It put all of my weight on a steel ring pressed against the bone on my inner thigh.

There was a bright side to this experience. My mother told the local butcher in Bulawayo, a Mr. Barnes, about my confinement. He came to see me one day. Before coming to Rhodesia, he had been a famous magician in England, known as Senrab the Magician. (Senrab was Barnes spelled backward.) He offered to teach me magic and visited often. Magic appealed to me. During the endless hours I spent by myself in bed, I became adept at manipulating small objects, making them disappear and then reappear. I think this may have given me some fine motor skills that later served me well as a surgeon. I remained friends with Mr. Barnes until I left Africa.

CHAPTER FOUR
SERONDELLA

During holidays, especially in the Rhodesian summer that began in October, my family lived at our vacation house in Chobe. The Chobe River is the major tributary of the Zambezi River, which forms the border between what were then Northern and Southern Rhodesia, now Zambia and Zimbabwe. The point where the Chobe joins the Zambezi is a junction of four countries. The countries' names have changed, but during my childhood to the north of the converging rivers was Northern Rhodesia, and to the south was Southern Rhodesia. On the west was the Bechuanaland Protectorate, later Botswana. Across the river from Bechuanaland was the Caprivi Strip, which used to belong to Southwest Africa. It is now part of Namibia. Smugglers and others who had an uncomfortable relationship with the law favored the area of closely mingled boundaries.

The forestry commission owned a large area south of the Chobe River, in Bechuanaland. This was wild country, unchanged for millennia. Wildlife including elephants, lions, and buffalo roamed freely. When the forestry commission left the area, the houses they had on the banks of the Chobe River went up for sale, and my parents and some of their friends bought them.

It was a two-day journey from Bulawayo to Chobe. We'd leave at dawn and drive all day to the Victoria Falls, a distance of about three hundred miles. The way was difficult, as it was a so-called strip road. Rather than pave the full width of two lanes in either direction, it was cheaper to build a single lane consisting of two parallel strips of tarmac on which your wheels traveled. To overtake another vehicle, you moved to the right, so that your left wheels remained on one strip as your right wheels careened over sand and gravel. The vehicle you were passing did the opposite, to the left. This was particularly hazardous when large trucks pulling trailers were involved, as the trailers swung wildly when making the transition from tarmac to dirt and back again. When a vehicle approached in the opposite direction, you each had to swing off to the left, the wheels on the right remaining on the strip. Driving halfway off the road raised thick clouds of dust, so that it was often difficult to see where you were going. Windshields were routinely cracked by flying pebbles. Accidents occurred frequently.

I remember a little gas station at Lupane, a town about halfway to the falls, where we liked to halt for a stretch to get gas. A black man in overalls pumped the gas by hand. It was a peaceful rest stop in those days. Years later the retired Catholic bishop of Bulawayo and a nun were shot dead in a guerilla ambush at Lupane.

It was hot. Our cars were not air-conditioned. The thin, brown African dust poured in through the windows and settled into every crevice of the car. The road was sometimes winding. Everyone grew a little carsick as the day went on. Herds of elephant or other animals crossing the road frequently forced us to stop. One of our friends was killed going to Chobe when he hit an eland at high speed. The large antelope weighed nearly a ton and had crashed through the windshield. Both the eland and driver were found several hours later with the bloody head of the antelope resting on the dead man's lap.

You could see the great plume of mist rising from the Victoria Falls when it was still twenty miles ahead—the "smoke that thunders," the Africans called it. We stopped there for the night, usually at one of the rest camps by the Zambezi River above the falls. The camps consisted of thatched *rondavels*, round huts with wooden doors and windows, containing camp beds. We made time to visit the statue of David Livingstone, the Scottish explorer and missionary who was the first white man to lay eyes on the falls. There were few tourists then, but the old colonial Victoria Falls Hotel existed largely for them. The Falls Hotel was too fancy and expensive for us. I much preferred the rest camps, anyway. You could watch hippos at play in the river, and sometimes elephants would wander through the camp in the evening on their way to drink.

In the morning, we crossed the Zambezi gorge over the spectacular Victoria Falls Bridge into Northern Rhodesia. The bridge's gleaming steel arch carried cars and trains more than four hundred feet above the river. It had been proposed by Cecil Rhodes as part of his grand scheme to link Cape Town to Cairo by rail, and though he died before the bridge was completed, it remains one of the great civil engineering achievements of the early twentieth century.

We drove to the town of Livingstone, where we picked up supplies. Heavy stores, such as forty-four-gallon drums of gasoline to run the boats, had been sent on ahead. After loading the car with groceries, enough for several weeks, we set off on a forty-mile drive over a dirt road that ran parallel to the north bank of the Zambezi. We were often halted by animals crossing the road on their way to the river. Eventually we left the main road, taking a small track that led to the river's edge. This brought us immediately across the river from Kasungula, in the easternmost part of Bechuanaland. There we unloaded the car and banged on an iron bar to signal the boats on the other side. Presently a small fleet of *makoros*, shallow canoes a foot or two wide and about twelve feet long that had been hollowed out from tree trunks, crossed the mile-wide river to collect us.

The boatmen, wearing ragged shorts but little else, stood barefoot at the back of each canoe with a long paddle, roughly carved from a tree branch, as we wove our way through the hippos in the water and the unseen crocodiles below. We sat on the floor of the *makoros* in puddles of water, careful not to move, as the sides of the boat cleared the water by about one inch and capsizing would have been all too easy.

An open truck waited for us on the other side. It was loaded by many willing hands. We rode in the back of the truck from Kasungula to Kasane, a small village that was the official border post ten miles on, though there was no real border at that time. This stop was a formality to let the authorities know that we had arrived in Bechuanaland. Kasane had a police post and an English district commissioner—a DC, as they were known—because Bechuanaland was a British protectorate at that time. There were fewer than a dozen inhabitants. Small whitewashed huts with thatched roofs served as offices and sleeping accommodations, and across the dirt track a two-person jail had been fashioned by putting a door on a hollowed-out baobab tree.

From Kasane it was another half day's drive in the truck over sandy roads through elephant country that brought us to the cottage we called Serondella. Though Chobe is now popular with German tourists dressed in expensive safari outfits, it was then one of the most remote and wildest ends of the Earth.

The house sat thirty feet above the river's edge, high enough to be safe from crocodiles and floods. The Chobe is a big river, in places some two hundred yards across. There were huge mahoganies and other shade trees near the water, and red bougainvillea climbed the walls of the cottage. Away from the river, the grasslands stretched toward the horizon, which was interrupted here and there by umbrella-like acacias.

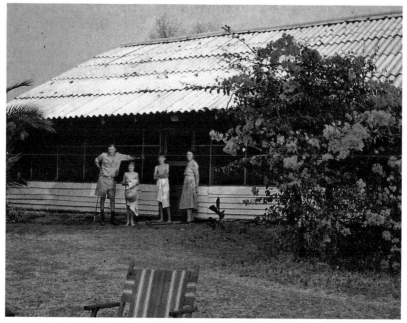

The cottage at Serondella.

Monkeys played on the corrugated iron roof of the house. It was a simple dwelling that had belonged to a forester. It had no electricity. There was a large, screened-in veranda that served as the living room and dining room, and several bedrooms inside. In the back was a kitchen with a wood-fired stove. The kitchen was always hot. We had a large water tank that was sometimes pushed over by elephants too lazy to go down to the river to drink. The water had to be boiled to make it drinkable. We stored it in canvas bags that were hung outside. Hot water was provided by a "Rhodesian boiler," a horizontal forty-four-gallon drum connected to the house plumbing and supported above an outdoor fireplace. It was a remarkably efficient system: the fire was lit half an hour before hot water was required. We had a houseboy named James who did the cooking and cleaning. The floors of the house were polished red cement. In the mornings, James would tie brushes to his feet and shuffle around the house singing.

There was game everywhere. Elephants came into the garden to eat the bananas off the trees, and lions prowled up and down the dusty track behind the house at night. Their grunting as they hunted kept us awake. The river was thick with hippos, sometimes submerged and other times peering serenely at us with just their eyes and ears above the water. Their distinct woofing in the evening signaled the cocktail hour for my parents. Hippos sound close by, even when they're not. As it got dark, we lit kerosene lamps and listened to the sounds of the bush coming alive in the night.

The boats were kept hauled out onto the riverbank in our absence. Relaunching them was a big job, as they were built of heavy teak and mahogany to make them harder for hippos to turn over. Our main fishing boat was a flat-bottomed barge. We would sit in the boat on deck chairs under an awning to protect us from the hot sun. We fished every day. The best times were in the early mornings or evenings, but we spent most of the day on the water, exploring the river or taking the boats to different parts of Chobe, where we would picnic and watch the animals. Though the north and south banks were in different countries, it didn't matter where we stopped. Nobody cared then. We had guns, but they were only for protection. We never shot anything, even for food.

We fished with spoon-type lures that had one side painted red and a six-inch hook trailing behind. We made these ourselves. We caught bream, for eating, and powerful, toothy tiger fish for fun. There were also two types of catfish. The *vundu* could be up to 120 pounds in size. It was not unusual for me to catch a fish larger than I was. Reeling in a big one could take an hour. Sometimes a fish eagle would swoop down and pick up a fish as we were bringing it in. Then there was a tug-of-war as the eagle rose into the sky, stripping most of the line off the reel until the bird realized it was hopeless and dropped the fish back into the water with a splash.

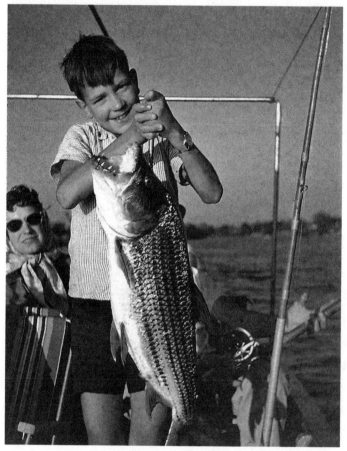

Me with a tigerfish at Chobe.

In later years it became possible to reach Serondella by car. Then we would go for drives along the riverbank in the evenings. This was hazardous and always exciting. Elephants, unaccustomed to humans, became outraged when their evening passage across the road for a drink at the river was interrupted.

They frequently made false charges at us, flapping their ears, stamping their feet, and throwing dust about while trumpeting loudly. We were never hurt, but the danger was real enough. Once, one of our neighbors went down to Kasane for the day in a truck and was forced to stop on the road coming home that night when elephants blocked the way. They surrounded the truck, one elephant pounding on the hood with her trunk. When the neighbor finally got back, he found that several Africans who had been riding in the back of the truck were no longer there. We mounted an expedition in the morning and returned to the spot. The Africans were discovered up in trees, cold and miserable but uninjured.

Some evenings after a day's fishing upriver we would rope the boats together and drift home as the sun set. It was peaceful and lovely, the water lapping at the boat as the river gently carried us along in the fading light. My parents would have their whiskey as we watched the elephants bathe in the river while giraffes, buffalo, and many kinds of antelope came down to drink.

To be safe in the bush, you had to know the rules and stick to them. We never swam in the river because of the crocodiles and always kept a wary eye out for them when close to the riverbank. We never walked out of the house at night because of the lions.

Even during the day, it was not safe to stray far from the house. Accidents did happen. There was a crusty old forester named Ledeboer who lived near Serondella and who boasted of being the only man in Africa to have been mauled by lions on three separate occasions. He'd survived, but at a cost, having lost an arm and a leg. His remaining hand had only two fingers. Actually, he couldn't blame the leg on a lion, as it had been taken off by a crocodile. Ledeboer didn't have many more parts to lose, but he was cheerful about it.

Crocodiles were an ever-present danger. Africans did their washing and bathing at the riverside in crescent-shaped enclosures constructed of logs set into the mud. Although this gave some protection, it was always possible for a crocodile to get onto the bank and then enter the enclosure or to take advantage of a loose log to force its way in. Late one night, an African brought the mangled body of a young boy to my father for help. The child had been taken by a crocodile while he was swimming, and his father had gone into the water to save him. There was a struggle until the father dug his fingers into the croc's eyes, and the boy was let go. Sadly, the child was dead by the time my father saw him. It wasn't unusual for visitors to seek medical help from my father. He always cared for anyone who was sick or injured. He never asked for anything in return, though maize or chickens were sometimes brought in as payment.

When I was about fourteen, I learned to water-ski. My parents would not have approved if they had known what I was doing. My brother and I devised a method using two boats that we thought was safe, and which most surely was not. One of us would get in the water with his skis alongside the chase boat. The ski boat would take off, and the chase boat would follow the skier. If he fell, he would be picked up immediately. The danger was an added incentive—we learned to ski quickly on the Chobe. I still remember skiing past sandbanks crowded with basking crocodiles, which slid into the water as I went by. I didn't know if they were startled or hungry. I eventually stopped letting Chris drive the chase boat because he would tease me by not picking me up right away and instead slowly circling and laughing.

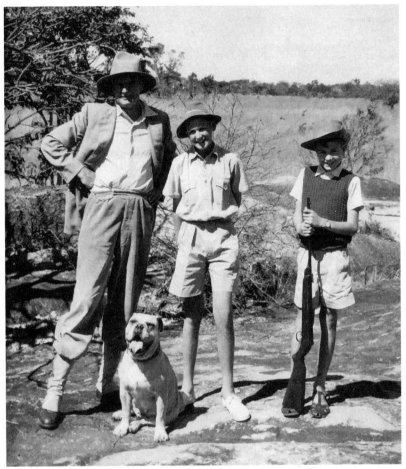

My father, my brother, Chris, and me with my dog, Annie.

My father had a great friend at Chobe named Pop Lamont. Pop had been a game ranger in the early days of the Kruger National Park in South Africa. This was before rangers used Land Rovers. While on patrol one morning, his horse was eaten from under him by lions. He managed to escape on foot while the lions busied themselves with the horse. When I knew him, he must have been in his seventies. He lived in a shack near the river with an African woman and her children. That they were his children was understood but never mentioned. He wore a big bush hat that covered his closely cropped gray hair. Pop almost never wore a shirt, and his sagging chest and back were like leather.

Pop had a maize field behind his shack that he protected fiercely. He kept an old rifle in his shack and an ancient shotgun that looked like a blunderbuss. One time Pop ran out of patience with a marauding elephant and shot it in his garden with the rifle. He cut off the tail as a memento. Soon the local Africans arrived with wheelbarrows to cut up the meat. When I went over there, they had cut a hole in the thick skin and were inside the abdomen, passing out morsels of liver, kidneys, and intestines to their families, who loaded it all into wheelbarrows.

Pop routinely fired off his shotgun at the baboons that were a constant nuisance. One day he told me that he'd hit one in the hindquarters and it had fled "doing the Twist." I was puzzled—I'd never heard of the Twist. When Pop explained that it was a dance popular with young people and the subject of a number of songs, I was surprised that *he* knew about it. Apparently he listened to his old radio at night when he had the batteries to power it. We had a radio, but it was seldom used other than by my father to listen to news and sporting events. I knew nothing about Western popular culture. I'd heard of Elvis Presley but had never listened to any of his music. Hearing Pop explain the Twist reminded me that there was a large world outside Africa about which I was utterly clueless.

Whenever we were at Serondella, my father would invite Pop for dinner. He would arrive around seven, walking to our house in the dark with a clean white shirt on, probably the only one he had. He wore pressed trousers and shined boots, and, of course, his hat. I think he felt obliged to dress for dinner as best he could. After the rest of us had gone to bed, my father and

Pop would sit up late into the night talking about the early days of Africa—meaning the early days of white people there. They smoked and drank whiskey by the light of a hurricane lamp while the insects beat against the veranda screens. A few always managed to get in, and they circled the smoky lamp casting moving shadows across the faces of the two men as they told stories. Pop looked forward to our visits. I think he was always sorry to see us go.

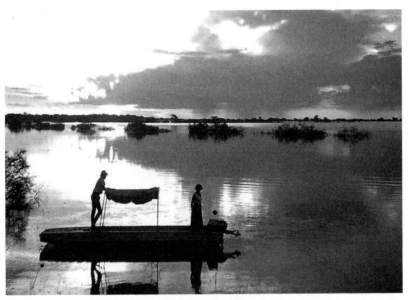

Sunset at Chobe.

Africans in the bush around Chobe often met with accidents, as they had beyond memory. The only white person I remember getting killed at Chobe was a man named Charles Trevor, who built the Chobe River Hotel in Kasane. Trevor and his wife, Ethnee, came to Kasane in 1959. Since there were few visitors then, a hotel had seemed a dubious enterprise. At first it consisted only of a cluster of huts, *rondavels* with thatched roofs. Originally an engineer, Trevor built a pontoon boat that could carry two cars or a truck across the river to keep the hotel supplied. The boat was fashioned from empty forty-four-gallon fuel drums fixed to a wooden deck. It was propelled by two outboard motors. This was for many years the only way a car or truck could get to Kasane from civilization, and it was a great boon to us as it permitted us to bring a car all the way to Serondella.

The hotel was just one of Trevor's unlikely schemes. He installed an old Studebaker engine on a paddle boat he called the *Chobe Belle*. He would ride in it up and down the river in the evenings, an African helmsman at the wheel. You could hear it coming a long way off. Trevor sat in a deck chair with a bitters-laced gin and tonic—pink gins, they were called—watching the elephants drinking along the shoreline as he cruised noisily past.

The first addition to the hotel was a bar, which opened on August 26, 1960, with a big party. All the white people in Kasane were invited. I still have the menu, which was signed by all twelve attendees, including my father. The others were local officials and a handful of guests staying at the lodge. Though I was there, I was not invited to lunch. I had just turned thirteen. I spent the day fishing from the bank of the river, waiting for my father so that we could travel the twenty miles upriver to Serondella before the dark made it too dangerous to be on the water.

Trevor was later killed while taking two women tourists up the river by boat. They had stopped on an island we called Crocodile Island for tea. One of the women walked a few steps from the shore and stumbled onto a nest of bees. African bees, known in Europe and America as killer bees, are fierce. When disturbed, they attack relentlessly. The bees descended on all three. The women survived by lying in the water and breathing through their straw bonnets. Trevor jumped into the water, too, but had to come up for air and was stung hundreds of times. He managed to get the visitors home by boat but then fell desperately ill. My father was the only doctor within two days' travel. I went along with him to Kasane as he looked in on Trevor daily. But there was no improvement, and Trevor was finally flown out of the bush to Bulawayo, where he died of kidney failure.

Trevor's wife had a son by a previous marriage, Robert Holmes à Court, who used to visit us at Chobe. He was in his early twenties, tall and lean, always with a taste for adventure. Robert owned an Aqua-Lung, and to our astonishment he would swim in the river with it. He must have come face-to-face with crocodiles many times. Perhaps they didn't know what to make of this strange underwater creature.

I remember a day when Robert threw eggs at some elephants to prove how close he could get. One elephant took exception to this treatment and managed to catch him. Trumpeting and shaking her great head, she tossed him several yards with her trunk. As he lay on the ground with his wind knocked out, the elephant tried to gore him. Robert held on to the tusks as she tossed her head trying to throw him in the air. Finally, he escaped by scrambling beneath her legs and into a bush. The elephant soon tired of searching for him and ambled off. Robert came away with only few broken ribs, which my father taped up while explaining how foolish the young man had been.

My best friend at Chobe was a man named Payeese, who was the chief of the local village across the river on the Caprivi Strip. He was also a witch doctor. A big black man with a long, curly black beard, he spoke no English and dressed only in a pair of torn khaki shorts. He wore a necklace of crocodile teeth. His own teeth had wide gaps between them, and some had been filed into points. Payeese visited us every day in his *makoro*, bringing fish he had netted. I spent many hours with him. He taught me how to make fishing nets and to paddle the *makoro* standing upright in the back.

Payeese gave me a steel-tipped fishing spear that I thought was the most marvelous thing I'd ever owned. One night I took it out in the shallows in a boat. My flashlight swept over the water and then caught a pair of eyes at the water's surface. There was a roar and a splash as the hippo exploded from the river and charged the boat. I threw the outboard into reverse, but it got stuck in the shallow water. As the hippo rushed at me, I tossed the flashlight away from the boat, and the hippo tore after it. When he realized I was still around, he turned to charge again. I managed to free the engine and escaped by inches.

Payeese was later killed by a hippo that overturned his canoe. I was devastated, and for a long time I had to remind myself every day that he wouldn't come paddling up to Serondella again. I still have two *karoses*, animal skin blankets made from a rare Bechuanaland antelope, which he gave to me.

....

When the Chobe was in flood every April, the fishing was bad. But one year the high water made the rapids between Kasungula and Kasane navigable, making it possible to reach Serondella by boat. Luis Preme, a man of all trades who lived in Kasane, picked us up in Kasungula, on the Northern Rhodesian side. We traveled in three boats up the river. The trip took most of the day, as we threaded our way through the unfamiliar rapids and the all-too-familiar hippos. I was in the last boat with a cache of stores and a delicate-looking female visitor from England, who was staying with us. An African who worked for Preme drove the boat. Halfway there, the engine quit. The boat drifted slowly backward downstream until it wedged itself in some rushes by the riverbank. A large crocodile slid into the water, and a few curious hippos popped their heads up to see what we were doing.

I wasn't especially worried. The driver and I both had plenty of experience getting balky outboards started again. But it was imperative that we do so. The other boats had gone on ahead and wouldn't have returned for us until the next day, since dark was approaching. After cleaning out the fuel line and the filter, I tried to start the engine and couldn't get it to catch. The African then tinkered with it a bit. After pulling on the start rope until he was tired, the man, who couldn't speak English, started shouting, "Bloody fucking thing, bloody fucking thing." As he heaved on the start rope one last time, the engine roared to life.

Our English visitor looked shocked by the language but was relieved to not be spending a night on the river. I asked the driver in Shona why he swore like that. "Swearing?" he said, apparently mystified. "Oh no," he said at last. "Those are the magic words Mr. Preme always says when the engine won't start."

Diamond smuggling was common in Chobe. I believed that Mr. Preme was involved in this illegal activity, because he once asked my father to take a packet of diamonds on our return to Bulawayo. My father refused. Webb, the superintendent of police, whose job it was to stamp out the illicit diamond trade, was also involved. I suspected my father knew Webb was implicated because of an exchange between them I once overheard at the bar in at the Chobe River Hotel. My father addressed him as Mr. Webb.

"My friends call me Webby," he answered, sounding annoyed.

"I know they do," said my dad.

I was shocked. I had never heard my father be rude to anyone. I asked him about it later, but he refused to discuss it. The law must have finally caught up with Webb, because he later shot himself in his office.

Life in Chobe sometimes owned a haphazard quality, as it did throughout southern Africa. Chance and fate were often in charge. In 1951, after they completed filming on the movie *The African Queen*, Humphrey Bogart and Katharine Hepburn visited Chobe. The DC escorted them. On the road outside Kasane, their vehicle was charged by a bull elephant. Though they were probably safe, the district commissioner shot the elephant there on the road and was celebrated for saving the life of Katharine Hepburn. The huge corpse lay on the road for months, a stinking mess. To go around it, a detour was made. The bend in the road near Kasane is still there, though few would remember how it came to be.

....

One year during the April floods at Chobe, when I was sixteen, my friend Richard Calder and I took a boat downriver on a fishing trip. An African drove the boat through the morning mist as Richard and I trolled. We stopped about two hours after dawn, having caught our breakfast. Nothing tastes better than fresh bream cooked over a campfire. We put ashore and started collecting firewood. I heard Richard call out to me. Something in his voice didn't sound right. When I found him he was bent over, reaching for a log but seemingly frozen in place. As I came closer, I saw why he wasn't moving. It was no log at all, but a huge snake, thicker than a man's arm. I could not see either end of it. Then it moved.

It was a black mamba, poised to strike. The black mamba is the deadliest snake in Africa. It can swim and travel on land faster than a man and can lift a third of its body off the ground to attack. Its bite is known as the "kiss of death," because it is always fatal. Death takes only minutes. The snake is actually gray, but the inside of its mouth is black. When a mamba is about to strike, it raises its head, opens its mouth, and sways.

The snake swayed slowly from side to side. Its unblinking eyes were fixed on us, its head some four feet off the ground. The open mouth was like a black pit, with two pale fangs exposed. Neither of us moved. I don't know why the snake didn't strike. After what seemed like an eternity, the mamba dropped its head, slithered off, and went down a hole in an abandoned termite hill twenty yards away.

Richard and I collapsed in the dust. It took a minute to recover. And then we went after it.

We were interested in snakes. In fact, we regularly collected snakes for the Bulawayo snake park, which paid by the foot—the rate depending on how long and how venomous the snake was. We knew a black mamba this size would be worth a small fortune. We knocked off the top off the anthill and poured a pint of petrol from the boat's engine down the hole. This had worked for us before, but nothing happened. Just as we were turning to get more petrol, the snake shot out of the hole. It looked at us, then took off in the opposite direction. I ran alongside it, beating the ground with a stick, trying to force it into the river. I had to run hard to keep up. The snake didn't hesitate at the water and began to swim across.

The river was about a quarter of a mile wide. We ran to the boat; Richard and I got in. The African refused to join us. We had reached the middle of the river when we caught up with the snake. We circled it, wondering what to do next. The snake tried to climb onto the boat. If it came to a choice between the crocodiles or sharing the boat with a black mamba, I was prepared to take my chances with the crocodiles. At the last moment, we managed to push the snake back into the river with an oar.

I fashioned a noose from some rope, attached it to the end of a fishing rod, and got it around the snake's head. We had it. Now all we had to do was get it back to Serondella and then to Bulawayo. We forced the mamba into a keep net we used for fish, and there it stayed, apparently safe.

No one was happy when we brought the mamba back to the house. Richard and I assured my parents that it would be impossible for it to escape. We put the keep net in a tin trunk and locked it. The mamba could go several weeks without water, and longer without food. From then on whenever there was a creak in the night, I would sit up in alarm, listening for a snake slithering through the rafters or a heavy *plop* as it dropped onto someone's bed.

When the time came for us to leave, my parents went ahead. I had my driving license, and we had come up in two cars, taking the ferry across the river. There was the problem of how to get the snake into Southern Rhodesia. We put the keep net into a large crate labeled "eggs" that we used when bringing supplies up from Bulawayo. If anyone at the border was so inquisitive as to open the crate, the inspection was likely to end then and there. As it turned out, we were waved through without any difficulty. We took the snake to the Bulawayo snake park. It measured fourteen feet long—the largest black mamba ever recorded. We were handsomely paid.

CHAPTER FIVE
IN THIS WAY YOU BECOME IMMORTAL

In early 1961, after finishing at Whitestone, I went on to Falcon College at the age of thirteen. Falcon had more students than Whitestone, around 250, and they came from all over central Africa. The school was in the bush thirty miles outside Bulawayo, on the site of a former gold mine called Bushtick. Mining had begun there in the 1920s and continued through the early 1950s. Eventually the gold played out and the shafts filled with water. Falcon opened in 1954 with an initial enrolment of thirty-four boys. The founders stated that they wanted the school to be "a place of dreams," from which its graduates would go on to achieve great things.

Essexvale, now Esigodini, was the nearest town, about ten miles away. Calling it a town was too generous. There was a gas station and a store that doubled as a pub. The countryside was the arid Matabeleland bush. The Essexvale estate was where Frederick Courteney Selous lived prior to the Second Matabele War, and where he returned in its aftermath.

When I was at Falcon, the classrooms, dormitories, and administrative offices were still the old mine buildings. The school houses were Tredgold, Hervey, Oates, and Founders—named for Rhodesia's early explorers and leaders. Tredgold, my house, was named after Sir Robert Tredgold, chief justice of Southern Rhodesia. While I was there, a fifth house was added—George Grey, a Southern Rhodesia pioneer who was killed by a lion.

Ten miles of rough dirt road led to the school from Essexvale. Inside the cattle gate at the main entrance, the road was lined with jacaranda trees that produced beautiful mauve flowers in the spring. These lingered through early summer. Then the flowers fell to the ground as summer progressed, carpeting the roads in blue. We had lush grass fields for rugby and cricket that were unusual in Rhodesia. They were irrigated with water from the flooded mine. The old slag heaps and open mine shafts were strictly out of bounds, though protected only slightly by straggly and rusted barbed-wire fencing. Naturally, we routinely explored these off-limits areas and were beaten for it when we got caught. Because Falcon was out in the true African bush, accidents happened more frequently than at Whitestone. One of the most common injuries was snakebite.

The school badge was a falcon with outstretched wings, and the school motto, *Sic Itur Ad Astra*, came from Virgil's *Aeneid*. It translates to "Thus you shall go to the stars." I believe Virgil meant, "In this way you become immortal." Falcon represented the remnants of colonial Southern Rhodesia. We wore blue blazers and turn of the century–style straw boaters on Sundays. On weekdays our uniform consisted of khaki shirts and shorts, with long socks and brown shoes or leather sandals. We dressed for dinner in "number ones," meaning long gray flannel trousers, white shirts, ties, blazers, and polished black shoes. Once a month, on a Sunday, we were given an *exeat*, Latin for "he may go out." The pass allowed us to leave the school grounds for a day. Since Chris and I lived locally, unlike most of the other schoolboys, we could go home and see our parents, though we had to be back at the school before nightfall. This was a big improvement over the long confinements at Whitestone.

We cleaned and polished the floors of the long dormitories and made our beds diligently. Morning and evening inspection was carried out by prefects—upperclassmen who had considerable authority over us. Prefects could administer beatings to younger boys, and there was no appeal if one took a disliking to you. One time when my brother, Chris, was a prefect, he ordered a friend of mine to cut the grass in front of Tredgold with a pair of nail clippers.

On Sundays, inspections were done by the housemaster. At inspection time, we stood at attention at the foot of our beds. Shirts and trousers were precisely folded on the small locker that separated one bed from another and held all our worldly goods. Our housemaster was a tough and burly, growling Afrikaner named Van Wyke. We called him Twikkie, or Twik. Twik said little. He taught physics and mathematics.

I had not been at Falcon long when, one evening, as we were standing at attention in the dorm, a loud boom reverberated across the campus. The windows rattled, and a bright flash lit up the night. The explosion had come from one of the nearby buildings. A sixteen-year-old boy named Dawson had been working on a homemade bomb. He had probably found the explosives discarded somewhere in the old mines. The device was a metal tube that had been between his legs when it went off. Though grievously injured and blinded in the explosion, Dawson remained conscious. The sister from the school clinic rushed to the scene but collapsed in tears when she saw the severity of Dawson's injuries. Smoking his habitual cigar, Hugh Cole, the headmaster, came down the road from his house to investigate. Dawson had been laid on the floor on a blanket.

"I know you are here, sir," Dawson said, "because I can smell your cigar. I'm sorry for the trouble." He died about thirty minutes later on the back seat of the headmaster's car, on the way to the hospital in Bulawayo. They cleaned up the blood the next day, repaired a hole in the roof, and picked up one of Dawson's fingers in the outside flower bed. No one knew why Dawson had been building a bomb, though it was agreed that he was probably just planning to set it off for fun.

The masters at Falcon were an odd lot, a mix of South African and English. It seemed the English in particular had come to Falcon as some sort of banishment, having failed at home or been judged temperamentally unsuited to teaching in a civilized country. One especially disagreeable man was a Latin teacher named Jenks, who walked with a limp, probably from an old war injury. Jenks was always dressed in a suit with a waistcoat, no matter how hot the weather. He was also a drunk. Most days he arrived at class wobbly. Sweating heavily and reeking of alcohol, Jenks was a tyrant. During one endless recitation, in which each student in turn read a page of *The Gallic Wars* by Julius Caesar and then translated it, he skipped my desk and went on to the next person. I was puzzled, because he had seemed to be looking right at me. When the last person had finished, he returned to me, and said, "Jamieson, who has avoided participation by the skillful use of camouflage, will recite the next page." Apparently he was so drunk he hadn't seen me.

I had my first girlfriend at Falcon. She was the daughter of the school's carpenter, an Afrikaner named Van Deventer. Her name was Vilma, short for Wilhelmina. She was an attractive girl, with smooth features, blue eyes, golden skin, and long blond hair. She was an object of desire and salacious speculation for every boy in the school. She chose me when we were both fifteen, and we started to see each other. The opportunity to meet was limited. I was invited to her parents' house for tea on Sundays, and afterward we went for walks together. I suspected that we were followed by a hundred eyes at a distance, so I was always on my best behavior. This was not what she wanted.

We sent our laundry in a pillowcase to the school's central laundry every week, and from there it went out to be cleaned. Every boy had a carefully memorized laundry mark, which had to be recorded on a list of what we sent in. Vilma's mother ran the laundry. She complained to Twik that the laundry lists were sometimes inaccurate. Twik summoned us to a house meeting and warned that a caning was in store for anybody who made a mistake in their laundry list in future. Mrs. Van Deventer would henceforth advise Twik each week as to any errors, though I don't think she knew this would result in beatings.

One week I was named. I was surprised, because I was certain my list was correct. I had checked and rechecked it. It turned out that Vilma had wanted to see me in the laundry room, and this was the excuse to get me over there. But Twik was informed and I got caned. I liked Vilma, but not that much. The relationship ended.

....

When I was sixteen, my father became ill. At first the only thing I noticed was that he was tired in the evenings and went to bed early, which was most uncharacteristic for him. What I didn't know what that he had developed leukemia. I think he tried to tell me that he was sick, but I was at a difficult age. He might not have wanted to trouble me, because I had important school examinations coming up. One of the lasting regrets of my life is that that neither he nor my mother told me that my father was terminally ill. There were so many things that I would have liked to say to him. Especially goodbye.

Because I was away at school most of the time, I never got to know my father as well as I would have liked. Once he took me on a medical safari into the bush to treat natives in remote villages, and I was in awe of the work he did. My most intense memories, though, were from Chobe, where he taught me how to fish and where to look for animals coming down to the river, smiling at me in his bush hat and smoking contentedly. When he was finally taken to hospital, my mother said I ought to visit him. I did, still unaware that he was dying. I found him in bed in the Bulawayo General Hospital, where my grandfather had died. I think he was in pain and probably medicated. We spoke about inconsequential things for a few minutes, and then he started talking about the staircase by the side of his bed. There was no staircase there. I was alarmed. A nurse came in and told me that I'd better go. I went into the hallway and wept. I never saw him again. He died a few weeks later.

There was a small, private funeral. We went to the local church at Hillside, and then my brother and I went out to the cemetery for the burial. My mother was too upset to go. A heavy feeling of loss washed over me when my father was in the ground. To this day I cannot attend funerals without anguish. A memorial service was held at Bulawayo's cathedral, which was filled to overflowing, probably for the first time in its history. Most of the people who came were black, which was unusual then. Many of them approached me after the service and shook my hand, saying what a great man my father was.

My father's death occurred just as momentous changes were taking place in Rhodesia. Within a couple of years, Ian Smith and his right-wing cabinet would declare independence from Britain, and Rhodesia would become an outlaw country. British sanctions were invoked and many things became scarce, particularly gas. Liquor was also hard to come by, and when Rhodesia started making an unusually strong alcohol from sugarcane, the joke was that you could buy a bottle and then decide whether to use it as fuel for your car or to get drunk.

Antigovernment activities, including terrorist raids against innocent white citizens, were on the increase. The government did its best to suppress reports of what was happening, and the newspapers became so heavily censored that their front pages were often half-full of blank spaces. I had been planning to go away to London for medical school for a long time. It had not occurred to me that I might not have a home to come back to. Now it did.

CHAPTER SIX
AN UNSPOILED LAND

Philip Henman was born in England, attended school there, and then went to Argentina to seek his fortune. He worked as a cowboy, or *gaucho*, on the Argentinean *pampas*, where he learned Spanish and became an expert horseman and skilled cattle rancher. In time, he moved to Rhodesia, where he bought Frederick Courteney Selous's ranch at Essexvale. His children were about the same age as me and my siblings, and our families had been friends for years. My sister, Margy, and Philip's daughter Jill shared a love of horses and spent many hours riding together. His son, David, a year younger than me, was my frequent companion.

Philip sold Essexvale and was appointed general manager of the Nuanetsi ranch, which, at two and a half million acres, was the largest cattle ranch in the world. You could drive for two days without leaving the property. The ranch had two centers of operation, the main headquarters in the south, and the northern headquarters, which were in a small town called Triangle, a hundred miles from the center of the ranch. Nuanetsi spanned an area from near the southern boundary of Rhodesia to Fort Victoria, halfway up the country. On its eastern flank, the ranch bordered Portuguese East Africa, now Mozambique.

I loved visiting Nuanetsi when I was growing up. But I was surprised and angry when two years after my father's death my mother married Philip, who'd lost his wife to brain cancer. I liked Philip, but I thought it was too soon for my mother to remarry and wondered silently how their relationship had come about. Nonetheless, I had a stepfather now, and from then on, when I was not in school, I spent most of my time at Nuanetsi.

The main house at the southern headquarters in which we lived had a large lawn. Like Serondella, it had a corrugated iron roof. I stayed in one of the guesthouses, which was made of mud mixed with straw and painted white. It had a thatched roof that made it cooler during the day. We took afternoon tea on the lawn under the shade of a tall tree. A semi-tame monkey called Jeremy stole sugar lumps from the tea table when no one was looking.

Philip insisted I always carry a gun for the walk from my quarters to the main house, as it was possible to come across a dangerous animal at any time. This caution was well founded. One morning a cook, carrying her baby on her back, went to the vegetable garden. It was in a fenced-in area near the river. She swung the gate open and started in without seeing the hippo that had somehow gotten inside the fence and was grazing on the vegetables. Caught off guard, the hippo charged toward the open gate, crashing over the cook and killing both her and the infant.

Despite being in the middle of the African bush, a hundred miles from the nearest town, we dressed for dinner and enjoyed elegant meals by candlelight. Electricity was supplied by a diesel generator, which only ran at night. The generator had to be started manually but was turned off from my parents' house by a switch on the wall. They would flicker the lights ten minutes before shutting down the generator to give all the managers time to light candles or kerosene lamps.

Nuanetsi was a vast paradise of unspoiled land with every kind of wildlife ranging free. People came from all over the world to hunt at Nuanetsi. It wasn't long before I felt completely at home there. I explored the ranch endlessly, usually on foot with a rifle in hand. One of my favorite places was about three hours' walk from the main house to a waterhole. A large baobab tree, which had been hollowed out by bushmen, stood beside the water. The room inside was twelve feet wide. I would sometimes stay the night inside the tree, sleeping on the ground next to a fire to keep lions away. In the cold dawn, as the sun climbed above the horizon, elephants, buffalo, zebra, giraffe, and many kinds of antelope emerged from the bush to drink. They stood together without fear, though when lions appeared only the elephants stayed. Knowing that this scene had been repeated every day of every year for many thousands of years warmed me in the morning chill.

A black man named Joni Fulamani was employed by the ranch to deal with troublesome lions and other animals that preyed on the cattle. Born in 1906, he was locally regarded as the greatest hunter and tracker who ever lived. Joni had worked at Nuanetsi since 1930. He had killed 120 lions, forty leopards, fifty-five hyenas, and hundreds of wild dogs—numbers that today would be appalling but that back then were a fact of life on a cattle ranch. Joni was in his fifties when I first knew him. Although I grew fond of Philip over time, it was Joni who really stood in for my late father when I came to live at Nuanetsi. I wanted to learn everything from him, and whenever I was at the ranch I spent as much time in the bush with Joni as I could.

Joni was humble, usually dressed only in khaki shorts and sandals. He had a stubbly beard that was going white. Although

Africans were not permitted to own guns, an exception was made for Joni, and he was never without his Lee-Enfield .303, an old British service rifle, and ten rounds of ammunition. I thought this gun was an inadequate weapon for dangerous game, though in Joni's hands that didn't seem to be the case.

Joni had scars that were a testament to his life in the bush. One day three lions killed six young purebred bulls, eating their fill before wandering off. Joni tracked the lions to a stand of trees, where they had decided to lie up and sleep off their meals as lions do in the heat of the day. He killed one with a shot to the head that woke up the other two. Joni wounded a second lion that disappeared into the bush. The other ran off.

Joni followed the wounded lion, a dangerous thing to do, but no hunter willingly leaves a wounded animal to die slowly. Joni picked up the blood trail and moved forward. The lion had flattened itself in a patch of tall grass, watching. As Joni came near, it seized him by the leg. Falling backward, Joni dropped his gun. He grasped the lion by the neck as it tried to bite his head. Joni nearly passed out as the big cat's hot, foul breath washed over him. Then Joni's dog, Setta, ran up and bit the lion on its hind leg. Roaring, the lion whirled on the dog, which jumped back. The lion turned back to Joni, clamping its jaws on his right arm. They struggled once more. Joni thought he was about to die when Setta again bit the lion from behind. The lion let go and hesitated for a moment. Joni managed to grab his rifle and shot it dead.

Another time Joni came to my stepfather to ask if he would pay for a new pair of sandals. Philip demanded to know why Joni thought that he ought to be responsible for buying his shoes. Joni apologized, explaining that his sandals had been damaged in the line of duty, holding up the mangled footwear. Philip asked him what had happened. Joni told us that he had caught a problem leopard in a steel leg-hold trap. When he approached the animal, it had broken free, tearing off half its leg, and charged him. Joni was knocked down but had been able to shove his right foot into the leopard's mouth. He used his left foot to fend off the claws that were trying to disembowel him. I had no trouble picturing all of this—Joni on his back parrying a leopard with his feet while coolly squirming close enough to his gun to grab it. I still have that leopard skin with its one short leg. And Joni got his new sandals.

We had a pet giraffe named Tiny, who came to the compound every evening to eat the banana leaves we fed her. She had long eyelashes and beautiful soft lips. We loved Tiny. Philip even forgave her for killing one of his prize bulls with a violent kick from her back legs. Tiny roamed wild during the day, and we became worried when she didn't turn up for a few months. Probably she'd been eaten by a lion, we thought. But then Tiny returned—with a calf, a perfect miniature of herself. We called the calf Tinier. Tinier never grew as tame as her mother. Some months later Tiny strangled herself in some telephone wires, and Tinier disappeared for good.

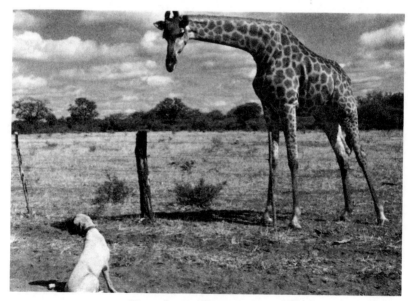

Tiny, the giraffe, with Annie.

We had two other pets that were an unusual pair—an ostrich and a zebra. The ostrich didn't have a name, but we called the zebra Waa Waa, after a funny neighing sound it made. They'd been raised together and were inseparable friends. We'd marvel as they walked side by side on the dusty road. One day the ostrich broke its leg trying to get into the vegetable garden through a fence. We did our best to patch up the injury, but the bird died the next morning. Waa Waa, bereft, stopped eating and died within a week.

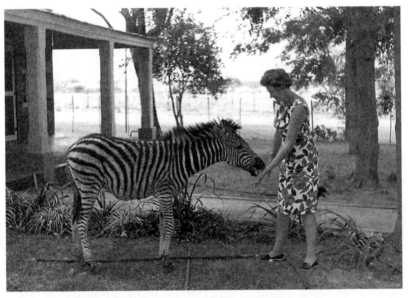

My mother with Waa Waa.

The office buildings and workshops where Philip worked were just over a mile from the house. There was a headstone on the lawn in front of his office, only steps from the entrance, that read, "On this spot in November 1956 the General Manager Mr. Dedman was killed by a buffalo." It was a reminder that in Africa danger could lurk right outside your front door.

The head mechanic was a black man named Butterfly. Butterfly could fix anything. He had a short, squat Land Rover built from parts cannibalized from other Land Rovers on the ranch. It was slow and had no brakes, windshield, or horn. Otherwise, it was perfectly serviceable. I appropriated Butterfly's car whenever I was at Nuanetsi. I learned to stop it by running over larger and larger bushes until it came to a halt.

Philip's desk had once belonged to Leander Starr Jameson. Imported from England when Jameson worked for Cecil Rhodes at the British South Africa Company in the late 1800s, it was made of mahogany, had a leather top, and was an altogether remarkable piece of furniture to find in this remote place. There was a walk-in safe behind the desk where an armory of guns of every sort was kept, mainly big-bore rifles for heavy game such as buffalo and elephant. My favorite was a .470 English-made double-barreled rifle. It had a kick that nearly knocked you over, but it could stop a charging elephant in its tracks. Although it afforded only two shots before reloading, in close encounters and dangerous situations, there is rarely time for even two shots anyway. And I figured that, knowing I had only two shots, I'd be more likely to make them count if I had to.

I had the .470 with me one day when Joni and I went after some lions that had gotten into an African-style thornbush *kraal* and carried away a calf. We tracked them deep into the bush and found a large male and three lionesses feeding lazily on the kill. As we approached, they lifted their heads and looked at us, nervously twitching their tails. We stopped about fifty feet away, stood still, and discussed the situation in whispers. We didn't want to kill all four. If we killed the male, we thought the others would leave. I shot the male between the eyes as he stared at me. His head dropped, and he didn't move again.

But the lionesses did not leave as expected. One of them took a few steps toward us. I shot her and started to reload. One of the other females then dropped her head and twitched her tail more urgently. This was bad. She grunted, took a couple of trotting steps in my direction, and then rushed forward in a full charge. While my gun was still open, she leaped at me from fifteen feet away. I heard the crack of Joni's .303. The lion tumbled forward through the air and landed on the ground dead, her head coming to rest by my toes. The remaining lion turned and ran off.

A cardinal rule in the bush is never to run from an animal. This is true for any predator and also applies to buffalo and elephant. The rule works for humans, too. Fear only encourages a coward and a bully. With animals, it is always best to stop and back away slowly, downwind if possible. Despite its size and ungainly appearance, an elephant can run twice as fast as a man. Elephants will generally stay away from you, but a female with a young calf or a bull elephant with a bad attitude is dangerous. We often came upon elephants while we were in the bush on foot. Most charges I experienced were "false charges." The elephant would run forward, flapping its ears and trumpeting, usually when taken unawares. After a few steps it would stop and back off, still trumpeting, stamping its feet, and flapping its ears.

The difficulty is that it's not always possible to distinguish a false charge from a real one. When an elephant tucks its trunk under its chest after lifting it up to sniff the air, and flattens its ears instead of flapping them in irritation, then it's the real thing and you are in trouble. If there is no escape and you have to shoot, the place to hit is just above the top wrinkle on the trunk to get to the brain. You will likely only have one shot.

I never had to shoot an elephant, and never wanted to. But I had another memorable close call not long after the day that Joni saved my life with the lions. We had a visitor from South Africa, a VIP with government connections. He'd come to the Nuanetsi to shoot a Cape buffalo, a formidable beast that can weigh more than two tons. It is the most dangerous of the big five game species—along with the rhino, elephant, lion, and leopard. In those days, more people in Africa were killed by hippos than any other animal—but more *hunters* were killed by buffalo. Joni and I were to guide the hunt. I wasn't impressed by the hunter—he was a young guy, about thirty-five—and I was even less happy with his gun, a .375 magnum that was fine for lions and leopards but which didn't have the stopping power for a buffalo you'd need in an emergency. But off we went, me with the big .470 and Joni, as always, with his .303.

We soon enough found a lone male buffalo. He was old and battered. Older males usually leave the herd and sometimes find the company of other retired males. This one seemed to be by himself. We tracked him downwind. When he was about seventy-five yards away, standing broadside to us, Joni tapped our guest on the shoulder, signaling him to take the shot. Everything looked good. The .375 would be more than enough for a heart-lung shot on a standing animal. I told our guest to aim a third of the way back from the front of the chest and a third of the way down from the top. If he was off in front, he'd break a shoulder. Too high and he'd break the spine. Either would put the buffalo down and make a second shot, if one were needed, easy.

The shot was low. I knew right away it was not a killing shot. The hollow thud of a low bullet striking is unmistakable. The buffalo galloped into a patch of brush and small trees. Joni and I glanced at each other in dismay. Nothing is more dangerous than a wounded buffalo in close cover. A Cape buffalo is the only animal that will stalk *you* when it's wounded, leaving a false trail or doubling back and lying in wait.

There was no thought of leaving the animal to die slowly. But rather than following up right away, I decided we should take the visitor back to the house. I wanted to tell Philip what was going on and to leave the man behind for his safety. The wounded buffalo would weaken from blood loss and begin to stiffen up, making him easier to deal with. Despite his protestations, we dropped off the visitor at the house and left a message for Philip. We were back where we'd last seen the buffalo about an hour later.

Joni, saying nothing, pointed to a few blades of bent-over grass and some frothy specks of blood. A lung shot. We looked at each other and started moving forward. The buffalo could be anywhere, including behind us. We tracked it for two hours. It was brutally hot. Sweat was running into my eyes. Around noon we came to a small rise with a thicket off to the right. The tracks continued straight ahead, but Joni stopped suddenly and caught his breath with a sharp hiss. In the same instant, a black shape broke from the bushes on our right. Joni fired. I knew he would not have missed, but his .303 did not even slow the buffalo. What came next seemed unfold in slow motion.

The horns of a Cape buffalo meet in a massive, impenetrable boss across the top of its head. When a charging buffalo lowers its head to gore you, this armor-like knot of horn makes a killing shot from straight on almost impossible. Not even the .470 could penetrate the boss. With Joni's shot ringing in my ears, I saw the buffalo coming at me at full gallop, his head up to see where he was going. Although the buffalo closed the distance between us in only seconds, it seemed a long time to me. I felt like I was watching this unfold, as if I weren't part of what was happening, and yet everything depended on me. There would be no second chance. It was a feeling I've since experienced in an operating room. I was calm. I raised my rifle and aimed at the buffalo's nose. He was close now, looming bigger by the instant. I fired, steadied the gun and found the second trigger, and fired again. I saw Joni step to his left. I moved right. The buffalo passed between us like a locomotive even as his legs began to fold under him. He skidded to a stop, dead, with two bullets in his brain.

I felt my heart begin to race then. Joni was completely composed. For him it was just another day in the bush. We returned home to find Philip waiting anxiously. The visitor on the veranda was having a beer. We went back to the buffalo so that photographs could be taken of the guest proudly posing behind it with his trusty .375.

....

One of my stepfather's ongoing projects was finding water for the cattle. The crocodile-infested Nuanetsi River ran through the ranch, and there was always water where the river was. But there were thousands of acres that were bone-dry. Water could be pumped from wells called boreholes, but it often had to be pumped long distances to where the cattle were. The pipes were buried, but no matter how deep they were put underground, elephants could always hear or smell the water and dug them up. Unlike lions or leopards, which killed the cattle and had to be hunted, elephants were more of a nuisance we put up with.

Philip and my mother had another house at the northern headquarters. It was closer to civilization. Local farmers sometimes came to hunt at Nuanetsi, but there were poachers, too, and we pursued them whenever we could. It was hard, because they usually hunted by flashlight at night. One time a woman phoned Philip wanting to get an urgent message to her husband. When Philip said he didn't know the man, the wife said, "Well, he is hunting on Nuanetsi." We found his car by the road, tracked him down, and took him to the police station. I expect he had a better time there than his wife did when he got home.

Much of Joni's time was devoted to tracking poachers. He taught me a lot about tracking. This was useful later on when poachers gave way to terrorists. Animals do not attempt to conceal their tracks—though buffalo may make false trails, especially if wounded. Humans breaking the law, however, often try to hide their tracks. Poachers would make false trails or try to confuse their tracks so you could not be sure how many of them there were. White poachers sometimes went barefoot instead of wearing shoes, hoping to be taken for natives. Other times they'd walk on the sides of their feet to avoid heel or toe marks or wore their shoes or sandals backward to make you think they were traveling in the opposite direction. Joni taught me how to tell if the track was from a man or a woman—or someone carrying a heavy load like a dead animal or a big weapon. He showed me the telltale signs that someone had been walking backward—the heel mark tended to be deeper than the mark made by the ball of the foot, the pace was shorter, and the feet were placed farther apart. Another trick poachers tried was to walk in a line and step in each other's tracks to make it appear as if there was only one of them. Sometimes a trail ended where the tracks had been swept away. We even came across tracks that had been partially obscured by the use of feet cut from hippos or elephants.

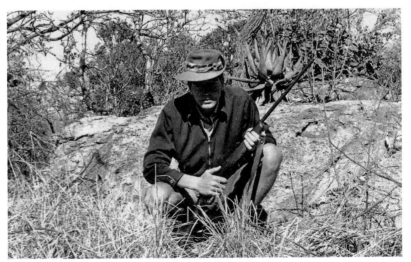

Tracking with Joni.

Joni saw everything: a patch of trampled grass, a few turned or broken leaves, stones or sticks that had been moved. He'd point to a track until I saw it and could tell him who or what had made it, and where it went. Every living thing that moved through the bush left marks on the land. Learning to read them was like learning a new language, one that had existed since long before there were words.

....

I had finished at Falcon and was living at Nuanetsi before going to England, where I was to attend medical school, when we received a troubling message from Falcon. David, Philip's son and my stepbrother, had disappeared. He was sixteen. He had told some friends he wasn't feeling well and was going to the sanitarium. He never arrived there. Apparently this hadn't worried anyone at first, as they waited two days before phoning Philip. I believe they thought David had run away and would just turn up again. But he hadn't.

I went to Falcon with Philip, Joni, and another tracker from the ranch, but the trail had gone cold. It was impossible to see where David had left the school grounds. His clothes and possessions in his school locker seemed undisturbed. We spent several days searching the bush around Falcon, looking for signs. We checked some of the mine shafts. But David had vanished. We agonized over whether he'd met with some kind of accident or had run off, a confused adolescent desperate to start life over somewhere else.

Philip never really got over the disappearance and presumed death of his only son. I missed him, too. It would have been much easier to accept had we only known what had happened to him. I think that Philip held out hope that one day David would just walk through the door. He never did.

PART TWO
THE CUTTING EDGE

CHAPTER SEVEN
LONDON

As British sanctions against Rhodesia grew harsher in my final years at Falcon, the civil war that had begun in 1964 deepened. After the Unilateral Declaration of Independence in 1965, Rhodesia was not recognized as a sovereign country, and factions within the revolt were being separately sponsored by the Soviet Union and China. It was a conflict with many faces. To many in the black majority, it was a war of liberation—though a significant number of blacks believed the war would destabilize the country and bring an end to a way of life that was preferable to what lay ahead. Competing rebel groups fought Rhodesian security forces and also each other. To whites shocked by atrocities committed in the name of freedom, the rebels appeared to be foreign-backed communists—or worse, a homicidal mob. And in time many events that could only be called acts of terrorism would unfold. This all played out against the backdrop of a country that was no longer functional. Money was in short supply under the sanctions, since it was all but impossible to get money in or out of the country. Rhodesia was coming apart.

And I was applying to medical school.

I was keen on going to London, which was the best place to train. I'd written to several medical schools requesting application materials and had been accepted by several programs. I decided on St. Mary's Hospital, which had been the first teaching hospital in London but was still smaller that most of the other schools. Many of the older hospitals, like St. Bartholomew's or St. Thomas's, where my brother had gone a year earlier, were opened as hospitals and only later took on medical students. I thought a smaller school would be an easier adjustment for me after a boarding school in the African bush. My acceptance letter arrived with a handsome color brochure showing scenes of student life at St. Mary's. I'd never seen anything like it.

Classes began in October 1966. I took the train from Bulawayo to Cape Town, saying goodbye to Philip and my mother on the long platform and then waving as the train chuffed and we began to roll beneath a coil of black smoke. The trip to Cape Town took three days. The carriages were grand—paneled in mahogany with green leather seats, the Rhodesian Railway "RR" emblem emblazoned everywhere. The train stopped often to take on water and coal. At each stop it was surrounded by vendors hawking trinkets and peanuts—which we called "monkey nuts." This was from an old game: You filled a jar with peanuts and then tied a string around its mouth and the other end to a tree where there was a monkey. Soon enough the monkey would come down, stick its hand in the jar, grab a fistful of nuts, and then be unable to extricate itself because it wouldn't let go. You then approached and the monkey ran around the tree as the string got shorter and shorter until the animal had pinned itself. You needed heavy gloves to catch the monkey and then let it go. Taming a wild monkey was out of the question. It was an odd amusement. Watching the peanut vendors on the train platform, the thought came to me that London would surely be different from everything I'd known until then.

The voyage from Cape Town to Southampton by boat took fourteen days. As we departed from Table Bay, many of the passengers threw streamers to people on the dock seeing them off. I wasn't saying goodbye to anyone, so I just watched. But as we steamed toward open water, I threw a coin in the bay, which was said to ensure that you would one day return. I made my way to steerage, deep in the bowels of the ship near the engine room, which throbbed day and night.

On the train from Southampton to London, I got my first look at England. It was shockingly green and, as it was autumn, much cooler than I was used to. In London I found my way to Wilson House, where new students stayed, on Sussex Gardens a few blocks from St. Mary's. My room was in the basement, but it had a small window and was warm and comfortable. I remember not long after my arrival walking to Hyde Park, which was nearby, wearing a coat for the first time in my life.

London felt like a different world. The brightly lit streets never got dark, which I found disorienting. Everywhere there were crowds of people and a cascade of noise that never ceased, even in the middle of the night. I wasn't accustomed to streets whizzing with traffic. I'd only glimpsed television and had never ridden an escalator. I'd come to London just weeks before a singing group called the Beatles would enter a studio to begin recording an album called *Sgt. Pepper's Lonely Hearts Club Band*, but I knew nothing about any of that. I was oblivious to "Swinging London" and the mod scene on Carnaby Street, and was content to stay that way. I had come there to become a doctor and had no thoughts of anything else.

St. Mary's was part of the University of London, founded in 1845 as a teaching hospital. Prince Albert laid the foundation stone. It was an immense brick edifice, with two ranks of arched granite colonnades flanking the main entrance. The entrance itself was curious, as there was a flight of steps up to the doorway—as there were at every other entry point to the building. I thought this was odd, as anyone arriving by ambulance would have to be jostled up the steps on a stretcher.

Although I was already admitted, I had to pay a formal call on the dean of the medical school, a man named Gordon Mitchell-Heggs. Befitting someone with that sort of double-barreled name, Mitchell-Heggs was formal in the extreme. He always wore a tailed morning coat with a waistcoat and striped trousers. His shoes gleamed. Although no one warned me ahead of time, he had two tests for admission. One was whether you opened the door for his secretary when you came in. The other was whether you caught the rugby ball he suddenly threw in your direction on your way out. I did both.

Sports were an important part of life at St. Mary's, especially rugby, which was thought to promote the kind of teamwork and selflessness that helped turn out good doctors. But it was in the field of medical research, notably immunology, that St. Mary's had made its reputation. In 1928, a St. Mary's researcher named Alexander Fleming discovered penicillin, revolutionizing the treatment of bacterial infections. On one of my first days, I discovered a plaque on Praed Street adjacent to the building where Fleming had worked commemorating the discovery. Later on, as a clinical student, I'd sleep nights in the room where Fleming had made his breakthrough.

I gradually accommodated myself to the clamor and cold of London, but one problem that didn't go away was my poverty. Rhodesian bank accounts were frozen under British sanctions, and I had little money. After paying my tuition, there was almost nothing left over. I earned extra money by waiting at tables at night, wearing an old set of tails that I had inherited from my father. I tutored the children of a few well-to-do families in the neighborhood who sometimes fed me, too.

English medical school was different from the American program, where you do a four-year undergraduate degree and then enter four more years of medical training. In England medical school was five years and you entered directly out of high school. After five years you were a medical doctor. If you wanted to do surgery, however, your training then continued. At St. Mary's we spent the first year and half of school mainly on the subjects that a premed student in America would study: chemistry, biology, anatomy. I found this crushingly boring. I was eager to begin learning medicine, impatient to be done with course work that seemed beside the point.

The exception was anatomy, which fascinated me. Gross anatomy—the dissection and close study of a human cadaver—is a long-standing medical school tradition. And it suited my aspirations to be a surgeon. Four students were assigned to a body, each of us partnered with one of the others. We started at one end of the body and finished at the other eighteen months later, carefully disassembling every muscle, ligament, bone, and organ, tracing the pathways of all the nerves and blood vessels. The bodies were embalmed in formalin, causing the anatomy room to smell vaguely of pickles. It took a while to get used to it. At the end of the day, the body was covered by a white plastic sheet, a partially disassembled former human waiting for us to resume.

In America, every medical school instructor is a professor. In England, only the head of a department is called professor. The professor of anatomy was a kind, elderly man named

Frank Goldby, who didn't say much except when delivering lectures, which he gave in a large auditorium. For some reason, Goldby always spoke directly to whoever was sitting at the end of the third row on the right-hand side. He never looked anywhere else. This was unnerving if you happened to be sitting there, and we soon learned to avoid that chair. Undeterred, Professor Goldby spoke to an empty chair day after day, until we decided to borrow a human skeleton nicknamed Fred from the dissection room. We put Fred in a lab coat and sat him at the end of the third row on the right. The entire class moved to the far side of the room, leaving Fred alone. Goldby came in, pulled out his notes, and without missing a beat delivered his lecture to the white-coated skeleton. When he finished, he said nothing, packed up his notes, and walked out as if nothing unusual had happened.

My partner in anatomy, and my closest friend, was Brian Jennings. He was a thoughtful, introspective person, smart and capable, and a bit of a renegade. I greatly enjoyed his company. Sometimes my parents would send me *biltong*, a dried, jerky-style game meat we used to eat in Africa. It was a rare treat for me. Brian asked to try some when I brought it for lunch one day to anatomy class. We'd been working on our cadaver for a while when I looked over and asked him how he liked the *biltong*. He looked at me oddly and said that it was horrible. It turned out he'd accidentally been chewing on a hunk of muscle we'd removed from the cadaver.

Brian and I sometimes put in extra study on Saturdays in the dissection room. We learned a lot in those quiet hours, a copy of *Gray's Anatomy* open on the body as we took our time cutting it apart. One Saturday, there was a commotion outside. Some local toughs were heckling a few of the female medical students. Brian called down, "Do you need a hand?"

"Yes, please!" one of the women answered.

Brian tossed down a hand from the nearest body. The street gang scattered. We later returned the hand to its owner.

The seemingly endless classroom work continued. I wasn't sure I'd made the right decision in coming to medical school. At night I'd lie awake thinking of African sunsets, when the dust in the air turned the horizon crimson. When you are near the equator, darkness comes on suddenly, without the gray twilight that lingered over soggy, gray London. In the bush you must be ready for the night, with wood gathered and a fire going before the sun is extinguished. A fire keeps lions and hyenas away and warms you under the soaring canopy of stars.

I missed my mother and Philip. I wondered what latest adventure Joni might have had. I don't think he would have liked London, with its trackless walkways and blaring streets. School was nothing like what I'd imagined. It was an unrelenting drudgery. We had no clinical work, no exposure to patients at all in the first year. My studies seemed unrelated to caring for actual human beings. I was frustrated and unhappy.

And then I got lucky.

Surgical teams in London hospitals consisted of two senior surgeons called consultants. Consultants were always addressed as Mister, a title that commanded respect. The consultants worked with at least two junior surgeons called registrars, who were the equivalent of American resident doctors. And then there were one or two housemen—interns, as they're called here. The whole team was called a firm and bore the names of consultants in charge.

The top firm at St. Mary's was the one run by Felix Eastcott and J. R. Kenyon. They did complex vascular surgery, which fascinated me, and Kenyon also did kidney transplants, which at the time were still considered pioneering. One day a houseman named Hutton from the Eastcott-Kenyon firm came down to the cafeteria, where I was having lunch and studying and wondering why I didn't just go back to Africa. Hutton happened to be from Rhodesia. He came directly over to our table and said that the firm was shorthanded that day and needed a volunteer to assist in the operating room. I don't know if he had me in mind, but I jumped up and told him I was ready.

I had never scrubbed in before, but it felt instantly right to me. They showed me how to scrub and how to get into a gown and gloves. I was not nervous but felt excited and had to remind myself to listen closely to any instructions I got and do precisely as I was told. The operating room—they call it the operating theatre in England—was brightly lit. The walls were tiled, the floor cement. The patient, a middle-aged man, was already on the table and draped in green surgical covers. The anesthetist, a guy named Knight, was sitting at the head of the operating table, dressed in a cap and mask but not a gown. He was reading a newspaper. This, I thought to myself, was a place where I wanted to be. It was quiet. The outside world seemed not to exist. Whatever routine concerns you were dealing with were left behind.

I felt something else, too: a solemnness that pervaded the room. Every OR is different. Some surgeons listen to music. Some crack jokes or gossip. Some, especially in England, rage and complain and throw instruments on the floor when things go wrong. But no one is ever disrespectful of the patient, who is accorded absolute dignity and deference. Unconscious, the patient has surrendered to the skill and judgment of a surgeon, the one person in charge of everything that is to happen. I remember the moment I stepped into that world.

The surgery was an abdominal sympathectomy, an operation not commonly performed now. It's a procedure in which a section of nerve near the spine is removed to improve blood flow to the lower extremities, the narrowed arteries often associated with diabetes or heavy smoking. The patient was on his back as Mr. Kenyon opened the abdomen. Without looking up, he told me to put my hand in and pull the intestines to one side so that he could locate the nerve. I reached into the wound and almost pulled my hand back in shock. It was warm! I'd of course had this experience gutting animals in Africa, but the only human body I'd put my hand into was a room-temperature cadaver.

From that moment on, I spent every spare moment in the operating theatre, scrubbed in and looking on, or sometimes up in the balcony watching from above. I always tried to watch Eastcott or Kenyon, whom everyone regarded as the best, but also because they were doing the kinds of pioneering surgery that most appealed to me. I also made it a point to watch St. Mary's most legendary surgeon, a man named Arthur Dickson Wright, whenever I could.

Dickson Wright, like most of the surgeons at St. Mary's, worked for the National Health Service (NHS), which paid for all of the hospital's regular patients. But he also maintained a lucrative private practice in the hospital's Lindo Wing, which was reserved for patients paying their own way. Even now, the Lindo Wing is considered among London's finest private hospitals, and the royal family routinely delivers its babies there. Dickson Wright performed more than thirty thousand surgeries in the Lindo Wing, where he also strong-armed wealthy patients into donating to St. Mary's.

Dickson Wright had begun his career before the discovery of antibiotics, in a time when you had to be fast and good. He was. Because he could get in and out quickly, and with minimal bruising and scarring, the risk of postoperative complications was reduced. Even though Dickson Wright had a reputation for being careless when scrubbing in, his patients almost never developed infections. And he had an uncanny ability to diagnose someone by just looking at them. His registrar would later confirm the diagnosis with whatever tests were needed, but Dickson Wright was never wrong.

When Dickson Wright turned sixty-five, he had been forced to retire from the NHS, but he continued his private practice. When I first saw him operate, he was in his early seventies. Watching Dickson Wright operate was like seeing the history of surgery playing out before your eyes. He was a throwback, the kind of surgeon that no longer existed, who performed every kind of operation. It didn't matter if it was a brain operation or an appendectomy, Dickson Wright could do it.

After I'd become a regular observer in the St. Mary's ORs, I discovered that I could learn a lot by watching the best—and also by seeing what could go wrong. I happened to be watching Dickson Wright on the day his career came to an abrupt end.

The patient was an older man having his prostate out, an operation Dickson Wright could probably do in his sleep. It involved opening the front of the lower abdomen. That day the anesthesiologist hadn't shown up. Tired of waiting, Dickson Wright decided to numb the man himself by administering an epidural at the base of his spine. He ordered the patient to roll over, stuck him, and then waited briefly before slicing him open.

Either the epidural was misplaced or perhaps Dickson Wright had been impatient, but as he made the incision the man began to writhe and moan in pain. The man's agony increased as Dickson Wright went on. After a few minutes, he yelled at the patient.

"Hold still!" he said. "You're not helping me at all."

Somehow the operation was completed and the traumatized patient was wheeled away to recover. The nurses from the

OR, horrified at what they'd seen, reported it to the hospital's administration. And that was the end of Dickson Wright, one of the best surgeons I ever saw, until he wasn't.

....

I was most interested in the heart. It's a remarkable organ. A pump made of muscle, consisting of four chambers and four valves, it beats about every second, day after day, year after year, for decades. Sometimes people are born with congenital defects in their hearts or acquire them as a result of some disease. Many others develop heart failure as a consequence of narrowing or blocked blood vessels that elevate blood pressure and overtax the heart—or suffer heart attacks when blood flow to the heart itself is interrupted. But as modern surgical techniques were developed to correct problems in every other organ of the body, the heart was left out. Unlike the other organs, the heart moves, a seemingly insurmountable barrier to operating on it. And if the heart stops, the patient dies. The heart is the body's on-off switch. No one dared touch it.

In 1896, a German surgeon repaired a stab wound to a man's heart, sewing it up as the heart beat on. The patient survived. And for the next half century, nobody tried anything like it again, though there had been some halting progress. During the Second World War, a US Army physician named Dwight Harken successfully operated on more than a hundred soldiers with severe chest wounds, including thirteen surgeries in which he removed shrapnel or bullets from inside the heart while the heart beat on and blood gushed from the incision. There were also a handful of risky repairs to defective valves, including an operation in which the surgeon used his finger instead of a knife to open up a narrowed valve. But the main problem remained: there was no way to safely stop the heart and work on it.

In the fall of 1952, a five-year old girl named Jacqueline Johnson was brought to the University of Minnesota Hospital in the States with a suspected hole in the entrance chamber of her heart. She was just my age at the time. She weighed less than thirty pounds and would surely die unless the hole could be closed. Dr. F. John Lewis, accustomed to the frigid cold of Minnesota—and perhaps aware that children sometimes survived near drownings when they fell through the ice in winter—decided to risk putting Johnson into a state of hypothermia and then stopping her heart long enough to sew up the hole. The theory—which had been tested on animals in the lab but never tried on a human—was that the cold would extend the time the brain could go without blood and be undamaged.

On September 2, 1952, with Johnson on the operating table in a shallow trough, Lewis administered the anesthesia himself, a mix of pentothal and curare. Johnson was then packed in ice, and her temperature began to fall. It took more than two hours for it to reach 28 degrees Centigrade—about 82.4 degrees Fahrenheit. Her heart rate, which had been speeding along at 120 beats per minute, fell below sixty. Lewis opened her chest and clamped off the heart, noting the time. Brain cells begin to die after four minutes without oxygen. How much longer hypothermia might extend that window was uncertain. Lewis made an incision in the right atrium and quickly found the hole. He sewed it shut as the clock reached four minutes. But it leaked. Lewis put in another stitch and it held. Five minutes had gone by.

Lewis closed the incision in the heart and removed the clamps. He began massaging the heart, which gradually returned to a normal rhythm. The chest was closed, and the ice was replaced with warm water. Eleven days later, Johnson went home, the first person in the world to have undergone open-heart surgery. Even though Jacqueline and I then lived on opposite sides of the earth, our paths would cross one day.

It was the beginning of a new age in surgery. The heart was no longer untouchable. But the risks of open-heart surgery remained staggering. After the Johnson case, Lewis operated on two more children with heart defects, using his hypothermia technique. Both died. Lewis stopped doing heart surgery and moved to Northwestern University. He retired to California at the age of sixty and wrote a caustic book, *So Your Doctor Recommended Surgery.*

One of the surgeons assisting Lewis when he operated on Jacqueline Johnson was his best friend, C. Walton Lillehei. After Lewis abandoned open-heart surgery under hypothermia, Walt Lillehei was determined to find a better technique. The ultimate goal was some sort of "bypass" machine that could circulate oxygenated blood through the body. This would allow the heart to be completely stopped and worked on not for a few minutes, but perhaps for hours. Experimental designs for a "heart-lung" machine had been tested as far back as the 1930s. None worked at first, but in March 1953 a surgeon named John Gibbon at Jefferson Hospital in Philadelphia repaired a simple hole in the heart of an eighteen-year-old woman named Cecelia Bavolek while she was attached to a primitive heart-lung machine. Gibbon had tried the machine once before, but that patient died. This time it worked, even though the blood clotted and foamed as it passed through the machine's oxygenator. But Gibbon's next five patients after Bavolek all died. He never used his machine again and quit heart surgery.

At the University of Minnesota, one of Lillehei's residents had a pregnant wife. One day he remarked to Lillehei that the

fetus was being kept alive by a kind of natural heart-lung machine—the placenta—and that it might be possible to connect
a child with a heart defect to a parent in order to make a surgical repair. It was a ghastly idea, but Lillehei was intrigued.
After trying the procedure on dogs in the laboratory—Lillehei
used a pump from a milking machine to move blood between
the animals—he decided to try it on a human.

When word got around the hospital about the procedure,
there was a chorus of objections. Nobody thought it was a good
idea. As one staff cardiologist put it, Lillehei was likely to kill
both parent and child and go down in history as the only surgeon to ever have a 200 percent mortality rate in a single operation. But Lillehei was undeterred, and on March 25, 1954, two
people scheduled for surgery were wheeled into the OR.

The patient was a thirteen-month-old boy with a ventricular
septal defect—a hole between the two main pumping chambers
of his heart. During the operation he would be connected to
his father, whose heart and lungs would keep both himself and
the boy alive while the child's heart was opened and the hole
repaired. Although the boy was certain to die without surgery,
losing the father would have been catastrophic, bordering on
criminal. "Whatever you do," Lillehei warned his team, "don't
take your eyes off the father."

Both father and son came through the operation. But the
boy died of pneumonia eleven days later. Still, Lillehei believed
he had demonstrated that the procedure—he called it "cross-circulation"—was sound. In the coming year, he performed forty-five open-heart surgeries on children using cross-circulation.
Twenty-eight survived and went home. Thirty years later all
but six of the survivors were still alive. The age of open heart
surgery that had tentatively begun with Jacqueline Johnson had
finally arrived.

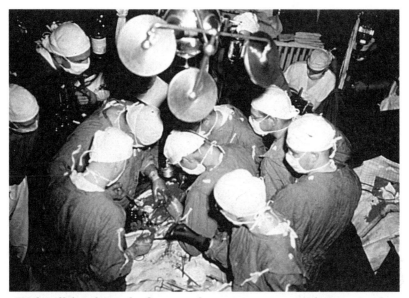

Walt Lillehei doing the first open-heart surgery case with cross-circulation. The father, acting as the heart-lung machine is on the right. Norman Shumway, my future boss, is on the far left.

Photograph courtesy of Dr. Lillehei

Gibbon's heart-lung machine was refined in the coming years, initially at the Mayo Clinic in Minnesota, and later by Walt Lillehei and his team at the University of Minnesota, who devised a "bubble oxygenator" that was simple and disposable. Lillehei used it in the OR for the first time in the spring of 1955. It would become the standard bypass machine for the next two decades.

Solving the problem of how to oxygenate the blood in a heart-lung machine was only one of a host of issues and open questions that had to be resolved. The machine also had to be able to heat the blood, because as it passes through the tubes and the machine it cools toward room temperature—which is much lower than body temperature. Eventually heart-lung machines would also be developed that could *chill* the blood for complex operations that involved both heart-lung bypass and hypothermia.

One question everyone wondered about was whether the continuous circulation of blood through the body at an even pressure would damage blood vessels. Normally, with the heart pumping, blood travels through the body in pulses and at different pressures—high pressure when it leaves the heart, and low pressure on the return. That's why your blood pressure is stated as two numbers, say, 120/75. Your arteries and veins have tone—that is, elasticity—to accommodate this pulsing river of blood. A person on the heart-lung machine has no pulse. As it turned out, this wasn't really a problem at all. The blood vessels tolerate the steady stream of blood from the heart-lung machine with no problem.

During the early days of repairing holes between the main pumping chambers (ventriculoseptal defects), the children and babies often suffered "heart block." The heart would not beat again after the surgery. The conduction system of the heart runs immediately below the hole that is the defect and is invisible. Particularly in those early days, when the sutures had to be placed hurriedly, and often with imperfect visibility, it was possible to place stitches around or into the nerves that made up the conduction tissue, and the heart would not beat again. The child would die unless connected to a pacemaker, and the pacemakers of the time were large machines, about the size of a lecture podium, on a cart that had to be plugged into the wall for their electrical power. The team made an extension cord one hundred yards long to transfer power from electrical outlet to electrical outlet on the long way back from the operating room to the patient's room.

On October 31, 1956, over Halloween, there was a large power outage affecting much of Minnesota and Wisconsin. One of Lillehei's young patients who was connected to one of the pacemakers died, since the electrical stimulus keeping the heart beating failed. This tragedy emphasized the defects of a system reliant on 110-volt electricity.

The very next day, Lillehei took the problem to a young technician at the hospital, Earl Bakken, who serviced the monitors, oscilloscopes, and other hospital equipment. Bakken was born in Minnesota in 1924 and since childhood had been fascinated by electricity and electronics. After the war, and having studied electrical engineering at the University of Minnesota, he started a company repairing medical electronic equipment with his brother-in-law, Palmer Hermundslie. The company was called Medtronic (MEDical elecTRONIC). The company was based in a small garage in Fridley, Minnesota, and got by (barely) by servicing the equipment mainly from the University of Minnesota Hospital.

Bakken found a circuit diagram for a metronome in the magazine *Popular Mechanics,* and within just four weeks he built the first transistorized pacemaker. He delivered this prototype to Lillehei for his opinion. Bakken continued to refine and test the handmade device in his garage and went back to the hospital to give one that could be used in patients to Lillehei. Much to Bakken's astonishment, when he came in the next day, he found the pacemaker already in use on a child. It was January 30, 1957.

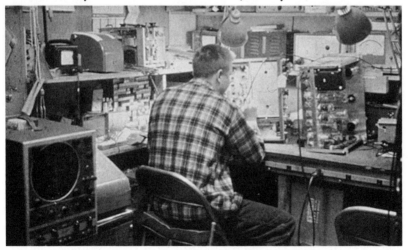

Earl Bakken in his garage repairing hospital equipment.
The very early days of Medtronic.
Photograph courtesy of Earl Bakken

Nowadays, of course, the regulation of medical devices through the Food and Drug Administration (FDA) would mean that a new device such as this could not be used in patients for years.

This was the birth of the first portable, wearable pacemaker. It was worn around the neck, like a necklace. Lillehei would later tell me how the children would often play with the knobs that controlled the device, which would have serious consequences! Technology continued to advance, however, and by 1960 Bakken had developed the first implantable pacemaker, with no wires going through the skin. Medtronic, which had struggled mightily in the early days just to pay the bills, would go on to become the world's largest medical electronic manufacturing company.

All of this work was taking place as I packed my tin trunk for Whitestone back in Africa. By the time I got to medical school, open-heart surgery had advanced considerably. So had organ transplantation. Kidney transplants had been done since 1950. The first liver transplant, by Thomas Starzl at Colorado General Hospital in Denver, happened in 1963, though it would be four more years before one of Starzl's liver-transplant patients survived at least a year. That left one milestone to be reached. As a medical student, I sometimes wondered idly if I might be the first surgeon to transplant a heart.

But on December 3, 1967, the world was stunned by the news that a young South African surgeon named Christiaan Barnard had performed a human heart transplant in Cape Town. Although Barnard had trained at the University of Minnesota under Walt Lillehei, no one outside a small circle of cardiac surgeons had ever heard of him—and none of them would have believed he was ready for such an operation. Everyone assumed the first transplant would have been done by either Norman Shumway at Stanford—another Lillehei disciple who had been scrupulously working out heart-transplant procedures in his lab—or Richard Lower at the Medical College of Virginia, who had worked with Shumway at Stanford. And in fact, Barnard had visited Lower and observed him do a heart transplant in a dog.

Now Barnard—handsome, charismatic, and seemingly hungry for celebrity—had come out of nowhere. His patient was a fifty-four-year-old grocer, Louis Washkansky, who suffered from diabetes and heart disease. Washkansky was in end-stage heart failure and had little to lose. And there was no shortage of donors in Cape Town, where people died in murders and car accidents all the time. South Africa was still rigidly segregated under its oppressive apartheid system. Barnard turned down a black donor, knowing the backlash it would have caused. Then on the afternoon of December 2, 1967, a young white woman, twenty-five-year-old Denise Darvall, was crossing the road with her mother to buy doughnuts. They were hit by a car, and the mother was killed outright. Denise suffered massive head injuries. Barnard had his donor. That night he called in his brother Marius, also a heart surgeon, and the rest of his team, and got to work. They finished just before six the next morning.

Even Barnard's own team had been caught off guard. As Marius later recalled, Barnard had done no research ahead of the operation to work out either the surgical procedure or the regimen of immunosuppressive drugs that would prevent rejection of the new heart. This was work that had consumed Shumway and Lower for years. Barnard simply skipped it.

Washkansky's initial recovery was spectacular. He began to breathe more easily and within a few days could feed himself. The world followed his every move. But Washkansky's second life was a short one. A shadow appeared on his chest X-ray. Barnard assumed this was caused by rejection and increased the immunosuppression regimen in the hope this would prevent Washkansky's body from destroying the new heart. But it wasn't rejection. It was pneumonia. The additional immuno-suppression allowed the infection to rage out of control. Washkansky died on the eighteenth day after the transplant.

But Washkansky's operation opened a logjam. Three days later, Adrian Kantrowitz of Brooklyn's Maimonides Medical Center transplanted a heart into a nineteen-day-old infant boy—who died six and a half hours later. As *Time* magazine reported in a cover story about Barnard on December 15, there were more than twenty medical centers around the world that had been working toward a transplant. At Stanford, Dr. Shumway had been ready to go a full month ahead of Barnard, but accidental deaths were relatively rare in Palo Alto, a university town, and he'd been unable to find a donor before his patient died in November. Shumway, widely regarded as the leader in heart transplant research, would have to wait until January 6, 1968, to do his first transplant. That year there were one hundred heart transplants done around the world. But results were so poor that by 1970 the number had dropped to eighteen. The only surgeon doing them successfully was Norman Shumway.

Barnard did a second transplant on January 2, 1968. The patient, a dentist named Philip Blaiberg, lived for nineteen months after the surgery. Barnard basked in his fame and was happy to be seen as a great pioneer. He never gave credit to the researchers in America who'd done the real work that made heart transplantation possible.

....

I was much closer to developments in the surgical treatment of vascular and heart problems that were taking place at St. Mary's. Felix Eastcott had come to St. Mary's as a medical student in 1936 and studied immunology and bacteriology under the legendary Alexander Fleming. Eastcott's real name was

Harry, but because he often stood with his hands clasped behind him like the cartoon character Felix the Cat, he'd gotten
a nickname that stuck. After graduating and going into surgery,
he had been a visiting resident at the Peter Bent Brigham Hospital in Boston, where they were working on the use of artificial
arterial grafts and also exploring the potential of kidney transplantation. One of Eastcott's mentors in Boston was Charles
Hufnagel, who later moved to Georgetown and teamed up with
a pulmonologist named Ken Moser, who was working out how
to operate on patients with pulmonary hypertension—high
blood pressure in the arteries that supply blood to the lungs.
This can be caused by a stenosis, or narrowing, of the artery
itself, or by the presence of blood clots in the lungs called pulmonary emboli. Blood backs up behind these obstructions.
The patient becomes short of breath and the heart fails as it la-
bors to pump blood against increasing pressure. Hufnagel—at
the urging of Moser—was the first to operate for this disease in
1961. Ken Moser took the procedure with him to the University
of California, San Diego, in 1968, when I was still a medical
student, and neither Moser nor I could have imagined that our
paths would cross one day.

The surgery to relieve pulmonary emboli was Hufnagel's
second breakthrough operation. In 1952, the same year that
Lewis did the first open-heart surgery on Jacqueline Johnson,
Hufnagel implanted the first artificial heart valve. It was a simple device—a hollow ball inside a tube that allowed blood to
flow in only one direction. Hufnagel designed it himself. It
was placed in the descending aorta of a thirty-year-old woman,
who did well after the surgery and resumed a normal life. The
one drawback was that the valve was noisy—the clattering ball
could be heard sliding up and down whenever the patient had
her mouth open. But it worked and the woman lived another
ten years before dying of an unrelated cause. Hufnagel's pro-

totype was so good that when I removed one from a patient thirty years after it had been implanted by Hufnagel, it was still working perfectly.

When Eastcott came back to St. Mary's, he teamed up with Charles Rob, the chair of surgery. Rob was a charismatic man who had been decorated as a lieutenant in the Second World War after he continued to operate on wounded soldiers after his leg was broken in a bomb blast. When Rob and Eastcott learned that Hufnagel had developed a procedure for freeze-drying blood vessels removed at autopsy for use in other people, they brought him to St. Mary's to show them how it was done. Alexander Fleming had just died. Eastcott and Hufnagel raided his laboratory for the equipment and set about creating a bank of frozen aortas.

Rob and Eastcott subsequently replaced many aortic aneurysms—enlargements of the vessel that causes the arterial wall to thin and weaken—with segments of these preserved human aortas called homografts. Homografts are structurally identical to the section of aorta being replaced, but because of the freeze-drying are no long living tissue. This was important because it meant the grafts would not be recognized by the recipient as foreign tissue—the critical step that initiates the process of rejection.

This was life-saving surgery. An aortic aneurysm is like a balloon being inflated to the bursting point. When an aortic aneurysm ruptures, the victim can bleed out in seconds.

Rob and Eastcott also performed the world's first carotid endarterectomy operation, in May 1954. It's a procedure to remove obstructing plaque from the inner wall of an artery going to the brain. This could only be done by stopping blood flow to the brain, and so hypothermia was used.

The patient was Mrs. Ada Tuckwell, a woman who was having repeated transient ischemic attacks—ministrokes. An angiogram had been taken in which contrast dye was injected into the suspect artery and then observed in a series of X-rays. This was itself a pioneering and hazardous procedure at the time. The angiogram showed a narrowing, or stenosis, of the left internal carotid artery that supplied the brain. Eastcott worried that the operation itself would result in a stroke. But everyone agreed that without surgery, Tuckwell would shortly have a crippling stroke anyway. Tuckwell was put under and packed in ice. Although the nurses' teeth were chattering, the all-day operation went well, and Tuckwell awoke without complications. She lived another twenty years, a period during which carotid endarterectomy became the most frequently performed vascular procedure in the world.

Rob eventually left for America, where he developed techniques for using veins to bypass arterial blockages that would later be essential in coronary bypass operations. Eastcott teamed up with Kenyon. They began using synthetic grafts instead of homografts to repair aortic aneurysms. These worked better than the homografts, which tended to dilate over time and form a new aneurysm.

The operation on Ada Tuckwell had been big news, though perhaps not as big a story as the one that broke a few days later when a St. Mary's medical student and track star named Roger Bannister broke the four-minute barrier in the mile. Bannister became a neurologist and was later one of my teachers.

....

As exciting as the vascular program was, I was even keener about work at St. Mary's on kidney transplantation. Dickson Wright had done what was probably the first in the world in 1949, when he sewed a kidney onto the arm of an elderly patient in a nursing home. The idea was that the kidney would do the dialysis that was failing in the patient's own kidneys.

But the graft never functioned, and because the procedure was gruesome, Dickson Wright never wrote it up.

The first recorded kidney transplant in Britain was done by Charles Rob at St. Mary's in 1955. The operation was on a young woman with kidney failure caused by sepsis—an often fatal condition in which an infection leads the body's immune system to overreact and attack its own organs. Nobody would do a kidney transplant in someone with sepsis today. The kidney failed, though it probably would have done so even without the complication of sepsis because of the unresolved issue of rejection. Rejection and how to suppress it was not well understood then. As it turns out, preventing rejection without killing the patient is the central problem in organ transplantation— one that I was eager to work on solving.

CHAPTER EIGHT
ANOTHER WORLD

Wilson House, my home as a student, was supervised by a retired naval captain named Gregory-Smith, who ran a tight ship. Though parking in London was scarce, some students had cars. A limited number of parking places in front of Wilson House were allocated to us. A medical student named Dalton had an old car that did not run. By virtue of his seniority, he had a parking place and somehow managed to leave his car in it. It never moved the whole time I lived there. This was a source of irritation to the captain. Every day he would say, "Dalton, when are you going to move that car?" It became a cause with him. I believe Dalton would have got rid of the car if it hadn't annoyed the captain so much. When Gregory-Smith retired, there was a big party. Dalton wasn't there. It transpired that Dalton had used the time to tow the decrepit car to the captain's newly purchased cottage in the country, where he left it in the driveway.

Almost everybody at St. Mary's was involved in rowing or rugby—or both. I played a little rugby, but it was rowing that

I liked. I was on the eight-man crew. At first I worried that the training—we rowed every evening on the Thames and worked in the weight room a couple of times a week—would get in the way of my studies. But I found that the workouts and the fitness actually made it easier for me to concentrate.

Every year we competed against the other London teaching hospitals. St. Mary's never lost. We also rowed at the big annual regatta at Henley, in Oxfordshire, that draws teams from all over the world. St. Mary's owned a country estate nearby that had once belonged to a family named Fleming. Ian Fleming, the creator of James Bond, had grown up in it. St. Mary's kept a few guest rooms in the old servants' quarters above the stables, and during the regatta they were given to us. One year we won our class at Henley. This made us eligible to join the Leander Club, an old boys' association for rowers that was considered a big honor. Members wore pink ties and socks. Unfortunately, there was an initiation fee that I couldn't afford.

The professor of surgery when I came to St. Mary's was a man named Bill Irvine. He was called Willie. Willie had a drinking problem. Everybody knew it. I used to go to watch him operate. It was unusual for him to be called in late, certainly after the cocktail hour, but I remember one evening when we had a leaking abdominal aneurysm, a serious emergency. Willie was summoned. When he arrived he was drunk. His registrar had to guide him through the operation, at times taking him by the hand to put a suture in the right place.

One time I'd been gone for a week to row in the regatta at Henley. When I got back, Willie asked where I'd been. When I told him, he sighed, "Ah," he said. "To be at Henley sitting on the lawn beneath a tent drinking champagne."

I also remember when a woman with a lump in her breast had come to see Willie. She was waiting for him in the examination room, having removed her top. Her husband was there with her. Willie came into the room, drunk, and stumbled forward. He caught himself by grabbing the woman's breast. The husband looked at me.

"Is he drunk?" the man asked. "IS HE DRUNK?"

I stared at the floor.

Eventually they fired Willie, a difficult thing to do to a professor.

The wards at St. Mary's were enormous, with tall windows and high ceilings. When the hospital was built, there was a theory that a large airspace helped reduce contagion. As we moved beyond our first years of medical school, these wards became our homes. The first things we learned were how to draw blood and how to take patient histories. Students rotated between different disciplines. Six months in obstetrics, followed by six months of internal medicine, and so on. When you were on the surgical rotation, you finished up your ward rounds by eight a.m. and then scrubbed in as a third or fourth assistant in the OR. You did little during a procedure, usually nothing more complicated than holding a retractor, sometimes for hours. Everyone ignored you unless the retractor moved.

When my surgical rotation came up, I was thrilled to be assigned to the Eastcott-Kenyon team, which was the most sought-after job. Eastcott was a legend, the most senior surgeon at St. Mary's. Always impeccably turned out in a three-piece suit, he was taciturn and unforgiving, an intimidating mentor. But if he got behind you, your career could take off.

Eventually, I became closer to Kenyon—a slightly rotund man who was as affable and pleasant as Eastcott was stand-offish. But I loved to watch Eastcott operate. He was precise and methodical, with no wasted moves. And he always worked in what surgeons call a clear field. When you cut someone, they bleed. But you can't see through blood, and so you can't operate unless you can stop the bleeding you've started. You have to tie off bleeding vessels and make sure you're not cutting anything unnecessarily. This blood-free "hemostasis" is essential. And Eastcott was good at achieving hemostasis. He always worked in a clear field.

It was good to watch these two talented surgeons work—because I really did little else but observe and stay out of the way. Eastcott and Kenyon still used the technique of total-body hypothermia for carotid endarterectomies when I was a medical student. One of my jobs was to get up in the dark of the early morning and haul blocks of ice up to the operating theater in a sack. It didn't take any skill, but I always made sure that I brought enough ice and got it there on time.

I rarely thought about anything other than my work as a medical student. I was friendly with the crew I rowed with and enjoyed the comradery. But I was always eager to get back to the hospital. Other than Brian Jennings, I didn't have any close friends. Brian knew another student named Hamish, whose family owned a cottage on Loch Duich, on the west coast of Scotland near the Isle of Skye. In the summer a group of us went up there on holiday. The scenery was spectacular. Loch Duich is an arm of the sea. In places it's flanked by mountains. It wasn't like Africa, but it was a refreshing break from grimy London.

One morning Brian took a small dory out on the loch by himself. He never came back. Later, we found the boat overturned with no sign of him. The weather was not bad, though squalls sometimes blew up quickly on the loch and he could have got into trouble. We reported Brian missing to the one policeman in the nearest village, and he helped us organize a search. But there was no trace of Brian. Hamish phoned Brian's parents. Of course, I thought of my stepbrother, David, and his disappearance. Brian was smart and sensitive, and medical school was demanding. Had he taken his own life? Gone off to take a new identity and start life over? There'd been no indication that he was upset about anything. It was a mystery. After a couple of days, we went back to London, taking our unanswered questions with us. Like David, Brian was never seen again.

....

In 1969, I was awarded the Anthony de Rothschild prize as St. Mary's most promising surgical student. Rothschild, the head of the Rothschild banking family, was a patron of St. Mary's, vice president of the medical school, and chairman of the board of governors from 1944 to 1957. He died in the Lindo Wing in 1961. His son, Evelyn—later Sir Evelyn—continued to support St. Mary's, as did Rothschild's widow, Yvonne. The Rothschild bank had funded Cecil Rhodes in the development of the British South Africa Company and the colonization of what became Rhodesia. The Rothschilds, whose family tree had branches extending across all of Europe, were one of the world's wealthiest families.

I was delighted with the prize, which I don't think had anything to do with my having come from Rhodesia. The Rothschilds had interests all over the world, and my background would have seemed ordinary to them. The prize included a cash award that I promptly spent to attend a meeting of the International Society for Transplantation in The Hague. There were thousands of people there, including many surgeons I had only read about. On my return to London, I was asked to write a report of the trip for St. Mary's. The report found its way to Yvonne Rothschild, who, to my surprise, took an interest in who had benefited from her late husband's generosity. Astonishingly, she asked to meet me.

This began a friendship that was to change my life over the next eight years. Yvonne was in her late sixties when I first met her. She spoke flawless English and French, as well as several other languages that I did not. She was lively and fascinating. Yvonne had fled France during World War II, hidden beneath a pile of hay in a horse cart. Now she lived at the family's vast estate at Ascott, in Buckinghamshire, about an hour's drive from London. Although Yvonne was Jewish, she was not observant and in fact loved to celebrate Christmas. To my amazement, I was invited that year. It would be the first of many holidays I spent with Yvonne.

I took the train up from London. I was met at the station by Hurley, the Rothschilds' butler—though he seemed to be much more like a chief of staff. I suppose Hurley was his last name, and I never found out his first. He took my tattered suitcase, put it in the back of a Rolls-Royce, and we were away.

The main house at Ascott was a Tudor-style mansion of two hundred rooms. It was the centerpiece of an estate that sprawled over more than three thousand acres. I loved to explore the magnificent gardens surrounding the house, thrilled to be out of the city. The gardens had been built by Anthony's father, Leopold de Rothschild, as a wedding present to his wife. There was a large greenhouse and a beautiful lake that had a swan on it. I later learned the swan had a nasty disposition and would attack you if you came too near. There was also a topiary sundial, and close by it a memorial to Anthony's brother, who had been killed in 1917 in the Battle of Mughar Ridge, fighting in Palestine against the Turks. Anthony had also been in the war and was wounded at Gallipoli.

Yvonne lived at Ascott with her mother, Sonia. The main house being far too big for them, they stayed instead in smaller quarters on the premises, in what they called "the cottage," though it was bigger than any house I'd ever been in. There was no question of me staying with them in the cottage, though there was plenty of room. It would have been improper.

So I was put in the main house and given free run of it. The house had a full staff by day, but in the evenings I was alone. It was incredible, filled with treasures. I remember a chess set in which the usual white and black pieces were instead made of solid silver and gold. I didn't know anything about fine furniture, which was everywhere, but I recognized the names on the many paintings hung throughout the house. Renoir. Cézanne. Gainsborough. My favorite spot was the library, which was lined with leather-bound books to the ceiling. It was huge—bigger than Raigmore.

I'd walk down to the cottage every evening for a formal dinner with Yvonne and Sonia. Naturally, I was expected to be in black tie. I had a dinner jacket and trousers that had belonged to my father. I had loaned them to my brother to wear to a rugby dinner that must have got out of hand as the evening wore on, and they were a little the worse for wear afterward. Chris admitted to me that he had torn the trousers crawling through a hedge. Hurley took them away to press before dinner, holding them at arm's length, saying, "I will do what I can, sir."

At dinner, Yvonne insisted that we speak French—a language I hadn't used much since Whitestone. She thought my accent was passable, though I understood the language far better than I could speak it. Meals at Ascott were always accompanied by wine, usually from the Rothschilds' Lafite or Mouton wineries in Bordeaux. I must not have realized that these were among the finest and most expensive wines in the world, as I usually asked for beer instead. Yvonne made sure I got my beer, though I suspected she disapproved. She did tell me that she was relieved that I didn't drink scotch. Apparently Winston Churchill had been a frequent guest when Anthony was alive and drank scotch all day long. Though he somehow never showed its effects at dinner, Yvonne wouldn't serve him good wine in the belief it would be wasted on his already overtaxed palate.

After dinner I'd walk back to the main house, where Hurley would let me in and then leave. He was back the next morning with my breakfast on a silver tray and a newspaper he'd ironed to take out the creases. Before he left he drew a bath for me, using a thermometer to ensure the correct temperature.

I took every chance to visit Ascott—holidays, weekends when I could get away. I came to love Yvonne, who was like a second mother to me when my real one was half a world away. Soon Ascott began to feel like home, which was strange when I thought about my actual home in the heart of Africa. Ascott was another world, but one I eagerly embraced. I was only mildly surprised when one day Yvonne said that she'd like to adopt me. She never did, of course, but if she had, it would not have changed the direction of my life.

Yvonne's son, Evelyn, would often appear for a short visit. He was always polite to me, though we never talked at length. I gathered that he was still something of a playboy then—into fast cars and racehorses. But he was also bright and accomplished. He ran the bank, eventually managed the queen's finances, and spent a number of years as the editor of *The Economist*. Evelyn always stopped in for at least a couple of hours at Christmas, the big event of the year. Christmas lunch was usually at Yvonne's daughter Renee's house, a horse farm in nearby Tyringham. Renee had married an Olympic equestrian named Peter Robeson. After lunch we would sit in the drawing room and listen to the queen's annual holiday speech.

Yvonne had a summer home in the south of France, in the mountains above Cannes. It was a converted abbey, and she sometimes took me there. We traveled by plane, invariably in coach—which I found amusing and endearing. The house and its gardens were lovely, and I could see the blue Mediterranean from my upstairs bedroom. We'd spend our days reading and relaxing. I always brought some work with me. Yvonne pointed out the driveway to the home of her nearest neighbor, Orson Welles. But I never saw him.

....

In my final years of medical school, I began to do temporary houseman jobs. This was an assignment given to senior students for a two-week period while an intern was ill or on leave. Although I had not yet graduated as a doctor, it was an accepted practice in a teaching hospital. To wear a long white coat and see patients and to be addressed as doctor was thrilling. I loved the work and rarely left the hospital. Medical students don't work so hard today, and I don't think they are nearly as single-minded about medicine. I don't know if this is ultimately good or bad, but I do know what they're missing: the passion that I felt coursing through me every minute that I spent becoming a doctor. I did not want to do anything else.

St. Mary's was especially nice late at night, when it was silent. I liked to stand by myself on the second-floor balcony and gaze down at the marble floor of the great entryway. Looking out into the dark space, I'd think how much I loved it, all of it, and how much I looked forward to the coming day, when footsteps would echo in the entryway and the hospital awakened and I could meet someone new who needed me.

CHAPTER NINE

IN THE BUSH
BENEATH THE
MOON

In the third year of medical school, we were granted a three-month elective, during which we were encouraged to work at another hospital or in some medically related endeavor to broaden our experience. Most people went overseas. I went back to Rhodesia.

I found a cheap air ticket on a charter plane, which left from Nice. I took a train from London. Having no money for a hotel, I slept at the airport. Every hour or so, a policeman would roust me and I would move on to find another place. I was not much rested when the plane left in the morning. It was a Dakota, a propeller plane with a range of little more than fifteen hundred miles. We stopped to refuel at Cairo, Khartoum, Entebbe, and Ndola, before finally arriving at Johannesburg. The trip took two days as we flew along just below the clouds, through stomach-turning turbulence in the heat of the day. Many passengers were airsick, which only amplified the misery onboard.

I left the airport and found my way to the outskirts of Johannesburg, where I stood on the side of the road with my suitcase, hoping to hitch a ride. The silence on the road outside the city was a welcome shock. Rhodesia was still fifteen hundred miles away. I rode with several Afrikans farmers who were interested in my experiences in England. Finally, I was left on the road on the south bank of the Limpopo. I walked across the bridge into Rhodesia, looking at the crocodiles basking on the sandbanks below. I was home.

I arrived late at night at the Elephant and Castle Motel, on the road from Beitbridge to Fort Victoria. The hotel belonged to the Nuanetsi ranch, but the drive from the headquarters, about seventy miles, was not safe at night. My mother and Philip arrived early in the morning to pick me up. At that point I still hadn't started doing any real clinical work at St. Mary's—I was still waiting to fall in love with medicine. Being back in Africa made me question everything again. I told Philip and my mother that I was thinking of not going back to medical school. Shrewdly, they told me to do whatever I wanted to. I had hoped they'd argue with me and that I could be stubborn. Instead, they'd made me think—something that more often leads to a good decision than does an argument. I realized that of course I would be going back to London.

After a few days at the ranch, I went up to Salisbury—now Harare—where my godfather had arranged for me to join the Department of Health. I was to embark on a medical safari to examine the native population. The department provided a Land Rover, two medical orderlies, and a native *ascari*, or policeman. The *ascari* usually accompanied the DCs on their trips into the bush, and he knew what he was about.

I drove, and the *ascari* and one orderly rode in the cab with me, the other orderly in the Land Rover's open back with the equipment. We covered about twenty or thirty miles each day, then set up camp. Somehow word went out that a medical officer had arrived, and in the morning there would be a long line for the clinic. Everyone in the village came out, and each, in turn, had to be seen. I was expected to prescribe something for everybody, as they would be humiliated to be sent off with nothing. Naturally, there wasn't anything wrong with most of the people I saw—the most common notation my orderly made in the record was NAD for "nothing abnormal discovered." Nonetheless, I'd hand over some aspirin or a skin ointment and call the next case.

Some people were sick, however, including a few that I could not help except to tell them to get to a hospital if possible. Snakebites were a common issue. In some cases the affected limb had gone gangrenous. There were traumatic injuries from accidents or encounters with animals. I saw several people with leprosy. And there were serious, sometimes advanced cancers. I saw one woman with a tumor on her jaw so large that she could not close her mouth. I also stopped in to examine a young man with what was surely one of the world's last cases of smallpox. He was covered in pustules. The villagers had wisely confined him alone in a hut, where he was being fed but was otherwise quarantined. I stayed on to care for him for several days. He survived.

Although unrest was spreading in Rhodesia, as yet it was not an all-out civil war. Most people still believed it would pass and Rhodesia would remain as it was. But there were certain places the *ascari* told me we could not go because it had become too dangerous. This was new. The dangers I'd grown up with had all been of the nonhuman variety.

These weeks were a remarkable interlude. By day I was a doctor—nobody I treated had any doubt. When we camped for the evening, I had little to do. I stretched my legs, washed, and changed, then had dinner, prepared by one of the orderlies, by the campfire. I would then make notes in my tent about the day's activities. I paid particular attention to the various eye ailments I observed. I later wrote this up and published my first paper on the occurrence of eye disease among African villagers.

....

I went back to the ranch before returning to England, where I decided to take off in an old Land Rover for some hunting. I was gone a couple of days. On my way back, I had a flat tire in a remote part of the ranch. The sun was going down, and a crescent moon had appeared. It would be dark in minutes. It was too late to look for wood for a fire. Camping until morning was out of the question. I didn't like the idea of spending the night in the Land Rover, so I started changing the tire. As I began I could hear the heavy coughing sounds of lions out hunting. They were close and downwind. They were coming closer.

To keep myself company, and to perhaps help warn the lions away, I turned on the Land Rover's shortwave radio. After dialing around for a moment, I picked up a news program. It turned out that the whole world was listening. Neil Armstrong and Buzz Aldrin were about to descend to the surface of the moon. As I looked around for a log to put under the Land Rover's jack, I kept one ear on the lions and one on the radio. Glancing up at the moon, I could not fathom how far apart these two events were—me changing a tire while being circled by lions in the African bush, and two Americans about to land on the moon. I was in a place that had changed little in thousands of years. They would soon step onto a place where no one had ever been.

I got the tire changed and sat for a while in the Land Rover, listening to the radio as moonlight filled the cab. The lions came up and sniffed around the vehicle but lost interest and left. I started the engine and headed for home, wanting to make sure I was back before Philip was worried enough to send out a search party.

I still had a little time left. I discussed my medical school decision again with Philip and my mother, who once again counseled that I should think it over and do as I pleased. Feeling unready to go back—but knowing that I would—I decided on a final camping trip into the bush. I headed for the eastern edge of the ranch, near the border with Portuguese East Africa. I made camp on a wide part of the Nuanetsi River that we called Buffalo Bend. At around two in the morning, I heard what I thought must be machine-gun fire in the distance. Only the army and the rebel terrorists had machine guns. At dawn, a Rhodesian Army Land Rover with three uniformed soldiers in it pulled into my camp. They told me they'd engaged a band of terrorists as they came across the border in the night. The rest of their outfit were now tracking them up. We talked for a while, and I offered them coffee. As they were getting back in their vehicle, we saw an unexploded hand grenade in the back—the type with a handle and what looked like a tin can on the end. Chinese made. Whoever threw it had forgotten to unscrew the base and pull the cord. As they left, one of the soldiers said with a smirk, "Well, I expect they'll get better at it." Unfortunately, they did.

....

It was time to go back to medical school. Had I not, my life would have been different, and not just because I'd left medicine.

One of the section managers at Nuanetsi was an old man named Mee. He lived with his wife in a small house on the ranch. I was friends with Mrs. Mee, who was always kind to me. She told me once that she and Mr. Mee had a close marriage. She would get up every morning at four and make tea, and then the two of them would talk until Mr. Mee left for work at five. One night after my visit, there was a knock on their door. When Mr. Mee went to see who it was, he was pushed back into the house at the muzzle of a gun. He was made to watch as his wife was raped, mutilated, and then killed. Then he was tortured and shot. The bodies were left on the lawn.

Eventually, it became too dangerous for my parents to remain at Nuanetsi. They left with only the clothes on their backs, telling nobody they were going. My mother had a handful of diamonds. She sewed them into the hem of her coat, and they headed for the border. She and Philip would have to live on those diamonds for the rest of their lives.

Rhodesia had become an idea that belonged to another era. In April of 1980, the country would rename itself Zimbabwe. But it had ceased to be the country I had grown up in long before then. As I watched from afar, first while I completed medical school and then as I began a career that eventually took me even farther away from Africa, the violent change that my father had feared swept over Rhodesia.

The civil war escalated. The Rhodesian economy collapsed. Bank accounts had long been frozen. Now other investments and property were seized by the rebels. In the coming years, a rampant inflation spun out of control. There was a saying, not far wrong, that if you stopped in a bar for a beer, your second one would cost twice as much as the first. The government kept printing money, sometimes running out of paper. At its peak in November 2008, the rate of inflation was incomprehensible, estimated at 6,500,000,000,000,000,000,000 percent. It became difficult to carry the number of notes needed to buy a loaf of bread. I still have a one-hundred-trillion-dollar Zimbabwe bank note printed in 2009. It's worthless.

Nuanetsi was appropriated without compensation by the new black government. It was handed over to the leader of one of the two rebel groups, Joshua Nkomo, who thus became the biggest private landowner in Africa. Nkomo had been a freedom fighter along with the current president of Zimbabwe, Robert Mugabe, who led a competing faction. It was an old story. Mugabe's people were Shona; Nkomo's Matabele. The two groups fought against the Rhodesian army, which was mostly black, and also against each other—as the Matabele and Shona had done forever. But now there was a twist. Mugabe was backed by the Chinese, Nkomo by the Russians. Like other struggles for independence in Africa, Rhodesia's war of liberation was also a Communist proxy war for influence on the continent. In May 1978, fifty civilians were killed in a clash between Communist militants and the Rhodesian army.

Nkomo's group was responsible for many atrocities. On September 3, 1978, they slaughtered a group of innocents in a way never seen before when they brought down an airliner with a Russian-made surface-to-air missile. The plane was on its way from Kariba to Salisbury, carrying fifty-six tourists on their way home from a holiday. Nkomo's men were hiding in the bush not far from the Kariba airport when they launched the missile. Eighteen people survived the crash when the plane came down in a clearing in the bush. Five of the survivors went to a local village to ask for help. Upon returning to the crash site, they heard voices and automatic gunfire. The other survivors were being killed, including women, children, and infants. A young flight attendant was shot as she tried to protect her passengers. A baby was bayoneted through the head. Nkomo's gang then looted the plane and the bodies. Three of the crash survivors who had remained at the aircraft avoided being killed by hiding in the bush. After a terrifying night in the cold, they were rescued by Rhodesian Army soldiers the next day, as were the five who had gone for help.

As horrific as this mindless act was, the response from the international community was almost as disturbing: silence. No elected leader, no country of the civilized or uncivilized world condemned the shoot-down and its blood-soaked aftermath. The lone voice of protest came from the Reverend John da Costa, the Anglican dean of Salisbury, who said from the pulpit, "This bestiality, worse than anything in recent history, stinks in the nostrils of heaven."

And then it happened again. Nkomo's group shot down a second airliner from Kariba on February 12, 1979. This time all fifty-nine civilians onboard died in the crash.

....

Zimbabwe today is a different country in more than name. Wildlife no longer roams free over private property. The mass slaughter of game animals by terrorists, poachers, and ordinary citizens faced with starvation has altered the nature of the bush. In Harare, a corrupt government continues to exploit and bankrupt its citizens. Little of what used to be still exists as it did. After I left Nuanetsi to return to medical school in 1969, I never saw the ranch again.

CHAPTER TEN
TIGER COUNTRY

Houseman jobs at St. Mary's were eagerly sought after. The top surgical position was with Eastcott and Kenyon. When I graduated in early 1971, I got it and began a six-month rotation with that firm. Running the service was left entirely to the two housemen. The other houseman was Mike Hampton. Theoretically we covered for each other every other night, but that is not how it worked out. After a day's operating, we worked late into the evening and then did ward rounds. After that, we had to get the patients ready for surgery the next day. We finished late each night and were always on call for our own patients.

One of the surgeries I got to perform early on was the removal of homografts, which were replaced with artificial grafts. I loved every minute and felt completely in my element. I had a room at the hospital, and all meals were provided. Although the total salary for the six months was less than $500, I had no expenses or outside responsibilities. I was as well off as I had ever been.

The hours were long. We never left the hospital. A lot was expected of us, especially from Eastcott. One night at around eleven p.m. I was on the mostly darkened ward checking on my patients. Through the shadows, I made out Mr. Eastcott by the door. I was not officially on duty, and I am not sure what he was doing in the hospital that late at night, but I went forward to greet him. As always, he was in a suit. I was in my white coat and white shirt.

"Ah," he said, "it's you, Jamieson. I didn't recognize you without your tie. I thought it was a boy from the village."

Eastcott was one of the court of examiners for the Royal College of Surgeons, which held exams twice a year, in the spring and in the autumn. The failure rate was about 80 percent. Eastcott once put his arm around a candidate who had done poorly and led him to a window overlooking a park. The trees had begun to leaf out after a long winter.

"Do you see those leaves?" Eastcott said.

"Oh, yes, sir."

"Well, then," said Eastcott, "come back again when those leaves fall off the tree."

Eastcott always wanted to be knighted, but he never reached this goal. You either had to be politically connected or have a successful outcome with a royal patient to get a knighthood. Eastcott came onto the ward one day announcing that he had a royal patient. We were advised to be on our best behavior. The patient was the nanny of the Duke of Kent, who was being admitted for treatment for varicose veins. Eastcott insisted that everything go without a hitch, particularly since the Duke of Kent himself would be bringing her to the hospital on Sunday afternoon so she could be worked up for surgery the next day.

I was in the hospital as usual that weekend. On Sunday morning Eastcott called me to say his elderly mother, who was staying with him at his home in Upper Harley Street, had fallen down the stairs and now had blood in her urine. He asked me to order an emergency intravenous pyelogram to inspect her kidneys, which I did. Shortly after that, I got a call from Southampton regarding a man with a leaking abdominal aneurysm. We were the national referral center for this life-threatening emergency. I told them to send us the patient at once and phoned Eastcott. He said he had just caught his finger in a deck chair while folding it up and told me to ask Barry Thomas, the registrar, to operate instead. I did this and then alerted the emergency room that Eastcott's mother would be coming in. The mere mention of Eastcott got everyone's attention. The emergency room doctor on duty that day was a temporary replacement who wasn't familiar with the emergency room staff or the way things worked in the hospital. He said he was just about to call me, because a boy had come in with acute appendicitis. Just about then Barry showed up to get ready for the aneurysm patient. We met in the emergency room and after examining the boy with appendicitis decided to operate right away.

While we were in the OR, the aneurysm patient arrived in the emergency department in extremis. They initiated a frantic series of blood transfusions and worked to revive him. In the middle of this chaos, the Duke of Kent—who should have gone to admissions—arrived with the nanny. As the duke stood there looking unconcerned about what was happening, the emergency room staff assumed that he must be Eastcott. The nanny was hustled off to radiology to have her kidneys looked at. The duke thought this was part of the normal preoperative workup for varicose veins.

Then Eastcott showed up.

He barged in front of everyone. As he waved his hands around, the staff noticed his bandaged finger. Thinking he had a minor injury and was nobody to be concerned with, they told him to sit down and wait his turn. Eventually it all got straightened out. I was happy to be unreachable in the OR as it was happening.

Eastcott never got his knighthood.

....

Eastcott had four daughters. If you were his houseman, you could expect to be called on from time to time to escort one of the daughters to some event. One day, Eastcott said that he had some tickets to the St. Mary's annual ball and asked me if I would like to go. Since I was too poor to buy my own tickets, I was absolutely delighted by his offer and accepted. "Good!" he said, "then you can take my daughter."

Despite what I'd heard, she was pleasant. We had an enjoyable evening. We did have to sit at Eastcott's table during dinner, which was awkward since I was technically his guest. I sat to the right of Mrs. Eastcott; he sat on her left. After dinner everybody got up to dance, leaving me and dour Mrs. Eastcott sitting at the table. I thought I should be a gentleman, and I asked her if she cared to dance. She replied crossly that she did not believe in that sort of frivolous nonsense.

Any thought I might have given to this evening causing Eastcott to see me in a more generous light disappeared with his next invitation. Eastcott asked me to come to his house for a dinner party. I replied that I would be honored.

"Fine," he said. "Come at six, and bring your white coat. You can serve the drinks."

Part of my job was to assist Eastcott with his private patients in the Lindo Wing. He also operated at the King Edward VII Hospital for Officers, and I helped him there, too. He would pick me up in his Jaguar. When we were done, he drove me back. Eastcott had a reputation for being miserly. He always seemed to have left his wallet behind when he invited the junior staff to the pub across the street after rounds. He never paid anyone for working with him on his private patients at weekends, as most of the other senior surgeons did with their housemen. So I was surprised when at the end of my six months he gave me a check for twenty pounds—at the time a magnificent sum to me. I showed the check around proudly until someone pointed out that it had not been signed.

This was a dilemma. With advice from my colleagues, I drafted a careful letter to Eastcott, in which I said that I was overwhelmed by his generosity and thoughtfulness but that he had forgotten to sign the check. I enclosed the check and said I'd be most grateful if he could remedy the oversight and send it back. I hoped this would end the matter. It did. The check never came back, and Eastcott never mentioned the letter.

Mr. Kenyon was more gregarious than his partner. Much as I admired Eastcott's talent, I found it easier to get along with Kenyon. One day he called to ask if I could fly to Greece with him and his anesthetist that evening. I dug out my passport, threw a few things into a bag, and rushed to the airport, where they were waiting. On arriving in Athens, we went to the hospital to see the patient, a shipping magnate who had an abdominal aortic aneurysm. The operation was scheduled for the next day. We left the hotel early in the morning. Since nobody in Greece had replaced an aortic aneurysm before, we had many visitors coming in and out of the operating room, some in street clothes. There was no air-conditioning and it was hot, so the windows were open. Flies buzzed around as we worked.

The operation went well, and I was assigned to stay with the patient that night. In the morning, the man's wife and family invited us onto his yacht. It was impressive, perhaps three hundred feet in length, with a full crew. We sailed to a private island to have a lunch at their villa. The boat had anchored a half mile off the beach, and the launch was put over to take us ashore. I decided to swim. I had only gone a hundred yards when I noticed that I was being accompanied by another boat from the yacht. I asked if there was a problem. One of the crewmen said that they were there to protect me from the "big fishes." The American Sixth Fleet was on station nearby, and garbage had been dumped from the large warships. This attracted sharks. At lunch I learned that there are forty-six different species of sharks in the Mediterranean, and that attacks do occur. I took the launch on the way back.

Some weeks later, when I was scrubbing for an operation, Kenyon came by and tucked an envelope into my back pocket. "The heavens have opened," he said. After I finished the surgery, I found a large sum of money in the envelope.

Of the body's great vessels, the aorta is primary. It's roughly the diameter of a large garden hose. It comes off the left ventricle—the heart's main pumping chamber—provides blood to the coronary arteries that supply the heart, and then ascends up and over the top of the heart in an arch before descending to take blood to the abdomen and lower extremities. The arteries that supply the upper body, including the head and arms, branch off from the aortic arch above the heart. Like the heart itself, this confluence of vital blood vessels is asymmetrical. On the left side, the left carotid and subclavian arteries come directly off the aorta and go to the head and arm. But on the right there is a single vessel, the brachiocephalic artery, which comes off the aorta for a short distance before branching into the right carotid and subclavian arteries.

I don't know if there is a seat of the soul. But if there is, I believe it is here, where the vessels that sustain the mind and the brain meet the aortic arch. To operate near the aortic arch is to operate in a dangerous realm—tiger country. One small mistake and the patient can transition to heaven quickly.

Eastcott had a patient, a forty-five-year-old man, with a stenosis in his brachiocephalic artery, the one that connects the aorta to the right carotid and subclavian arteries. Eastcott was out of town when the man went into distress, so Kenyon decided to operate. I scrubbed in to assist.

Kenyon opened the chest, just to the right of the sternum, and exposed the artery. Something happened, and it started to bleed. In almost the same instant, a tear near the juncture with the aorta appeared and immediately began extending downward into the aorta, like a zipper opening, disappearing beneath the sternum and out of reach. Blood gushed from the chest with each fading heartbeat and splashed to the floor. Kenyon kept working, but it was hopeless. In twenty seconds the patient was dead. The operating room went silent. We all looked at each other in disbelief. I'd never seen someone die on the operating table before.

Tiger country.

When I completed my six months with Eastcott and Kenyon, I moved on to the second six-month rotation, this one in general medicine, which would complete my year of internship. I went to the Royal Lancaster Infirmary, where I worked with a doctor named Adamson. Lancaster, in the west of England, north of Blackpool, was a nice place to live. Adamson saw a lot of cardiac patients. Watching many of them die in the intensive care unit convinced me that there must be better ways to care for people with critical coronary disease. Being treated in intensive care did not seem to have any predictive value as to who would get better and who would not. Coronary-artery surgery was in its infancy then. In 1971, only two hundred coronary-artery bypasses were done in the whole of England. If you had a heart attack or bad angina, the treatment was medical, involving drugs, which helped to alleviate pain but did nothing to alter the patient's outcome.

The nursing staff at Lancaster was spotty. Some were great, and a few were terrible. One day a senior nurse came to me and complained there was a patient refusing to take his medication. I went to see the patient, who was propped up in bed with a cold tray of breakfast in front of him. He looked asleep, so I shook him. He fell over. He must have been dead for some time, because his fingers and arm were already stiff from rigor mortis.

If a patient died and was to be cremated, you had to sign a form saying that there was no need for any further investigation or autopsy before the body could be disposed of—paperwork for which you were paid two and a half pounds. This was a lot of money to a houseman. We called it ash cash. It was enough to fill up my car with a tank of gas. I had a Triumph Spitfire, which I had bought new. From the moment I drove it home, it had made a knocking sound from the rear wheels. I suspected it was one of the bearings, but every time I took it back to the dealer, he said he couldn't hear anything. I eventually traded that car for a Triumph TR7 at the same dealership. The dealer took the Spitfire for a test run. When he came back, he asked, "What's that knocking sound coming from the back?" I told him I couldn't hear anything.

CHAPTER ELEVEN
THE DIFFICULTY
OF NOT SELF

I was a doctor now, but not yet a surgeon. I still had to complete my general surgery rotations, which would take another four years. This would include heart surgery, which I looked forward to. I also had to do six months of trauma and emergency work. And, most daunting of all, I had to take the first part of the Fellowship of the Royal College of Surgeons examination. In those days, to pursue a specialty like heart surgery, you had to do a full residency of general surgery first. That meant you had to be a Fellow of the Royal College of Surgeons—your FRCS being the final step.

The examination was in two parts. The "primary" FRCS was an exhaustive test on anatomy, physiology, and pathology. The anatomy section was particularly difficult. The standard textbook was *Gray's Anatomy*, written by Henry Gray in 1858, updated continually ever since, and running to more than two thousand pages. We had to memorize each one.

The primary FRCS exam was customarily taken about two years after the house jobs. It was an essay exam in which you had to write on three subjects over three hours. The subjects were often obscure. I'll never forget one that I got: vesico-vaginal fistula, which is an abnormal connection between the vagina and the bladder. Most physicians would go a lifetime without ever seeing a case.

If you passed the written examination, you went on to the oral portion, which was even more intimidating. You spent an entire day answering questions from two-person teams of examiners, again on the subjects of anatomy, physiology, and pathology. There was no latitude for wrong answers. The pass rate for the primary FRCS was between 10 and 15 percent. Once you got past that hurdle, it was back to clinical work for two or three more years until you accumulated the experience necessary to take the final FRCS.

The final FRCS was a three-day obstacle course of written examinations, followed by oral examinations if you passed the written part. The oral portion usually involved examining actual patients, making diagnoses, and discussing treatment options. Most of the examiners were well-known surgeons, and it was prudent to know who they were and to be able to quote from books they had written.

At the end, everyone gathered at the bottom of a staircase in the great hall of the Royal College of Surgeons. If you passed you were called up to the balcony, where your name was checked against the list. Then you joined the examiners in an oak-paneled room where they were drinking sherry. From that point forward, your title was no longer Doctor, but Mister. This tradition goes back to the days of Charles I, when surgeons were not physicians but barbers—hence the Mister. But now to be called Mister is a great honor.

....

In 1968, two years into medical school, I had approached the chief of pathology at St. Mary's, Ken Porter, about working in his lab. Porter wore glasses, had black hair, and worked in a small office adjacent to his lab that was zealously guarded by his secretary. Porter was studying immunosuppressive drugs, which were essential to overcoming rejection, the major problem in organ transplantation. He worked closely with Tom Starzl, the American surgeon who was pioneering liver transplants. Starzl sent tissue samples from failed or biopsied organs to Porter, who studied what happened in the rejection process. Porter was the world's leading authority on rejection, how it happened, and how it might be controlled. Porter was generous with me and let me have research space in his lab.

When someone gets an organ transplant from another person, the body's immune system recognizes that it does not belong, but is instead foreign, or "not self." This protective mechanism helps you get rid of bacteria, viruses, and even some early cancer cells that are not meant to be there. This is why we usually survive a cold or other infection. When an organ is transplanted to replace one that has failed, the body will also do its best to get rid of the transplant.

Porter knew that there are two types of rejection. One involves lymphocytes, white blood cells that destroy the organ. The other process is driven by antibodies in the bloodstream that destroy the blood vessels supplying the organ. Lymphocytes can cause rejection in a matter of days, whereas antibody-caused rejection may happen quickly or take months or even years. Porter noticed that in kidney transplants, after two or three years, atheromas developed—a hardening of the arteries supplying blood to the kidneys. Porter wanted me to look at this type of rejection. Soon I was interested in heart transplantation and started doing experiments in which I'd implant a rat with another rat heart alongside the existing heart and connect it to the blood supply so that it would beat, even though it was not a working heart. You could feel this transplanted heart directly through the abdomen. I did lots of tests, but I could always tell how the heart was doing just by feeling it.

We tried many drugs, mostly on rats. Because rats are so commonly used in research, you can get inbred strains that are essentially identical twins. So if I transplanted a heart from an A strain of rat into another A, it would not be rejected. But if I transplanted from A to B—a different strain—the heart would be rejected. Interestingly enough, I also discovered that if I transplanted a heart from A to B, and then back again into another A, it would also be rejected. That was because the heart picked up all kinds of cells from B—so-called passenger cells.

I met every week with Porter's pathology group. At one point he suggested that I wasn't cut out for surgery, that I was too "sensitive." I think what he meant, but was too circumspect to say directly, was that I was too thoughtful to be a surgeon. There was prevailing view then that surgeons weren't as bright, that they were more like mechanics than doctors. But I was determined to become a surgeon, and in the end Porter was supportive.

During my general surgery rotation, I continued to work with Porter. By now he had moved into a new research facility. Porter was one of the first to use electron microscopy to explore the process of organ rejection. The device occupied most of an entire floor of the building and could produce a magnification of ten million times actual size.

I had my own office and an assistant. And Porter paid me, which was most generous. Whenever I had time, usually at night and on weekends, I was in the lab doing heart transplants in rats. I was still studying the rejection process itself, something that even today is not completely understood. But my real goal was to figure out how to prevent rejection by modifying the body's response to foreign tissue. Finding drugs that could depress the immune system wasn't hard. The trick was to figure out the fine balance between too much and too little. Too much immuno-suppression and the patient cannot ward off ordinary infections. Too little and the transplant will be rejected. In the early day of trial and error, this was as much art as science.

But for me it had a special appeal, because I wanted to do heart transplants. If you transplant a kidney and it's rejected, the patient can go on dialysis and live until a new kidney can be found. But when a heart is rejected, life can end quickly.

Eventually I focused on a process called "hyperacute" rejection, in which organ rejection takes place not over the course of days, but within minutes. This reaction occurs when the body has been pre-sensitized, meaning that it has preexisting antibodies to the transplanted organ. Such antibodies are present when a patient has already had a transplant, or multiple blood transfusions from different people. There are also preexisting antibodies that will attack organs transplanted from other blood types and from other species. I reasoned that drugs that could control hyperacute rejection, which happened fast, would also work on more ordinary, slower rejections. And there was the tantalizing possibility that if you could prevent hyperacute rejection, it might be possible to use transplants from other species—pigs, for example. A major difficulty with organ transplantation is finding enough donors. If animals could become donors, it would change everything.

My first scientific papers—aside from my survey of eye disease in Africa—were published in 1974, on the subject of hyperacute rejection. I used guinea pig hearts transplanted into rats. The hearts were rejected within minutes. The electron microscope showed that the blood clotted within the blood vessels, starving the heart of oxygen and stopping it. This kind of rejection was so severe that nothing could prevent it. In the years since I did those early experiments, little progress has been made in modifying this type of rejection. Though it is now possible to create genetically modified pigs to make their organs seem more human when they are transplanted, cross-species transplants are still not possible. Stanford's Norman Shumway was famous for his thoughts on the subject. "Cross-species transplantation is in the future," Shumway said, "and always will be."

I was still finishing up my requirements for the FRCS. I spent six months as casualty officer at St. Mary's, doing emergency medicine. This was usually routine, as we were in central London. Severe traffic accidents from the motorways would go more often to the suburban hospitals. Two cases do stick in my mind. Late one night we received a young man who had had a motorcycle accident. The gas tank between his legs had ruptured, covering him in gasoline, which then ignited. When he was brought in, his clothing and flesh were still smoking. I tried to remove his boots and trousers, but most of his flesh and skin came, too. This was beyond what we could treat. I transferred him to a burn hospital, where he soon died. I was scolded for sending them a hopeless case.

On another occasion, a man had been working under his car when the jack slipped. The car came down on his face. They were able to remove him, but his face was completely destroyed, a mess of jellylike flesh. Somehow his forehead and brain had been spared, and he was still conscious and trying to talk. The moving mass of flesh below his brow was like a horror movie. He was accompanied in the ambulance by his girlfriend, who was hysterical. She showed me a photograph of how he used to look, asking to have him put back that way, which was of course out of the question. We eventually got him out of hospital, but he looked different from the way he used to.

Mostly we dealt with cuts and bruises and the odd knife wound. Unlike American emergency room doctors, we never saw gunshot wounds. The pubs in Paddington had last orders at eleven p.m. and closed at 11:10. That gave time for the locals to finish their drinks, pick a fight, get beaten up, and be brought to the hospital. We would get busy at around eleven forty-five p.m.

I did a general surgery rotation at Northwick Park Hospital, just outside London, and then came back to St. Mary's one final time to work as a registrar on the surgical unit, where the professor of surgery at the time was Hugh Dudley. Dudley was fifty-one when I worked for him. He always wore a white coat with short sleeves, a unique uniform. He had an interesting background. He studied in Edinburgh, followed that with a fellowship in Boston, and was appointed senior lecturer in the Department of Surgery at Aberdeen University. He had a bright future, but he made an abrupt move to Australia to take up the first chair of surgery at Monash University in Melbourne. The move to the other side of the world was probably precipitated by the scandal that erupted after he shot his neighbor's dog for being a nuisance. He'd come back to Britain, to St. Mary's, in 1973.

Dudley was widely published in medical journals, which is undoubtedly how he got the job. He was a poor surgeon, a pedant, and a terrible bully. As his registrar, I was his designated whipping boy. Though I am sure he had some good qualities, I thought him a tyrant.

One of my main jobs was to accompany Dudley on morning rounds, which started at seven a.m. Normally this would be easy work, but Dudley had a habit of asking for obscure blood test results that seemed to have no relevance to the patient at hand. I had to review every patient's chart ahead of time, which meant that I had to start rounds at five a.m. I tried to think of the rigid discipline of my boarding school days, but it didn't help much. I was on my guard from the start. On my first day, I had knocked on Dudley's door for rounds at two minutes past seven. "Come in," he said, and looked at his watch. "I said seven a.m., not two minutes past." I told him I would do better in the future.

Dudley's senior registrar, one step up from me, was Peter Fielding, who served as a buffer between me and Dudley when things got particularly bad. Peter, who was a much better surgeon than Dudley, taught me a lot about general surgery. One morning, after I had been working all night without rest or sleep, I had to help Dudley do one of his strange and complicated operations. I wondered why he was doing it so awkwardly. I had never seen this method before. Of course, I didn't dare to say anything. After an hour or two, he realized he had sewn everything backward. You might imagine that he would have been embarrassed about it, but no. He considered it entirely my fault for not stopping him.

I refused to call Dudley at night when an uncomplicated emergency case came in. It was easier—and in my view better for the patient—for me to deal with it myself. This eventually got me in trouble.

Dudley had an elaborate way of doing a bowel anastomosis, a surgery in which a portion of the bowel that is blocked is removed, and the ends are then sewn together. Dudley's suturing, which was absurdly complex, often fell apart after a few days. Because this could be dire for the patient, he invariably took the additional step of making a small incision above the repair and then temporarily diverting the bowel out through the abdomen, where a colostomy bag collected feces. After the original repair was healed, he put the bowel together again.

I thought this was a terrible thing to do to the patient, and also unnecessary if you did the anastomoses correctly. I'd seen Fielding repair a bowel with a much less complicated technique that seemed almost always to work and did not result in a colostomy bag. But Dudley insisted I do it his way, which I had to do when he was around. At night, it was a different story.

On rounds one day, Dudley happened to read the operative report of a bowel case I had done two nights before. He was outraged that I had not used his method. He told me that if I ever did it again, I would be fired. But I ignored this, and shortly thereafter a woman with a bowel obstruction came in in the middle of the night. I did it my way, thinking this time I would have to make sure the patient was discharged before Dudley had a chance to read the operative report. But Dudley unexpectedly showed up early for rounds. I knew I was about to be dismissed.

I quickly explained the situation to Fielding, who was sympathetic. Dudley's routine was to spend about ten or fifteen minutes on each patient, asking questions, making an examination, and then discussing the case with students. During this time the curtains around the bed were drawn. While Dudley was attending to a patient, Fielding slipped out and enlisted a couple of nurses to help shuffle several patients around so that my bowel case was at the end of the ward where Dudley had begun rounds. Dudley thought he had already seen her. I lived to fight another day.

My last recollection of Dudley is from December 1976. I had a wisdom tooth that was causing me great difficulty. A dentist removed it along with some of the bone in my jaw. My face was so swollen I couldn't talk, and I missed three days of work. Dudley thought this was inappropriate and refused to pay me for the whole month.

CHAPTER TWELVE
A MATTER OF LIFE AND DEATH

The University of Minnesota was the center of the cardiac surgery universe in the States. In Europe it was the Brompton Hospital in London. Founded during the reign of Queen Victoria, the Brompton was first hospital in the world to specialize in diseases of the chest—in those days mainly tuberculosis, the most common cause of death then. Tuberculosis afflicted people without regard to social status, though poor nutrition put people at greater risk. One in two hundred people developed the disease, and half of those died within five years. Originally called the Hospital for Consumption and Diseases of the Chest, it eventually became the Brompton, named after the part of Chelsea where it was located. Its long wards were named for British royalty.

In the early days, the Brompton was run by physicians, not surgeons, since there was no surgical treatment for tuberculosis except in the late stages of the disease. When I first went to the

Brompton in 1973, the buildings were much as they had been for 130 years. But the surgeons had come into their own.

In February 1935, a Brompton surgeon named Arthur Tudor Edwards did the first complete removal of a lung in Europe, a pneumonectomy. Another chest surgeon, Clement Price-Thomas, later joined Arthur Tudor Edwards at the Brompton. On September 23, 1951, Price-Thomas removed the left lung of King George VI, Queen Elizabeth's father. A heavy smoker, as most people were in those days, the king had been ailing for some time. The king did not go to the hospital; the hospital went to the king. The operation was done at Buckingham Palace. I later learned from someone who assisted on the operation that when Price-Thomas went out to tell the queen about the surgery, she asked if she could see the king. "Not now, Your Majesty," was the reply, "my assistants are still closing his chest."

Winston Churchill, who was a confidant of the king and was to become prime minister again the following month, was present. He asked, somewhat indignantly, "Mr. Price-Thomas, you do not close the king's chest yourself?"

"Mr. Churchill," Price-Thomas said calmly, "I haven't closed a chest in twenty years and do not intend to start practicing on the king!"

Clement Price-Thomas received a knighthood for operating upon King George VI, becoming Sir Clement. Apparently, nobody ever told His Majesty that he had cancer, as he was puzzled until he died as to why he was not improving. Price-Thomas, having chain-smoked throughout his life, even while seeing patients, eventually got lung cancer himself.

I joined the staff at the Brompton as a senior house officer, an SHO. In most hospitals, an SHO would not have to have the Fellowship of the Royal College of Surgeons to be appointed, but competition at the Brompton for these jobs was so fierce that generally this was required. Even an SHO would generally be a Mister. I did not yet have the fellowship but thought I would apply anyway. At my interview, I sat down before Mr. Matt Paneth, one of the Brompton's senior surgeons. He only asked me one question.

"Are you married, Jamieson?"

"No, sir," I said.

I got the job.

I was assigned to spend the next three months with Chris Lincoln and Stuart Lennox, consultant surgeons who worked with Paneth. Though he was in his forties, Lincoln had only just been made a consultant. He did all types of adult pulmonary and cardiac surgery but specialized in pediatrics. On my first bewildering day, I was introduced to one of the registrars, Ibrahim Mustafa. Mustafa was from Nigeria and had a gentle disposition. The only cardiac surgery I'd done until then had been in rats. I couldn't wait to get started.

Mustafa took me around to see the patients. Among them were many small babies who had had heart surgery. Just twenty years after Lewis and Lillehei performed the first open-heart surgeries in the world, operations to repair complex defects were done every day at the Brompton. I was fascinated by the machines, monitors, and chest tubes coming out of the patients connected to bottles by the bedside to drain blood after the operation. Catheters in the bladder collected urine to monitor kidney output—a good measure of how a patient is doing. When the cardiac function drops, blood flow to the kidneys slows, and urine production decreases as a result. It's one symptom of the body's protective response to a lower cardiac output, as it prioritizes blood flow to vital organs such as the brain. This makes the hands and feet cold to the touch. I was fascinated to see a standard thermometer taped to the big toe of the babies. The temperature was recorded at ten-minute intervals. One of the first signs of impending trouble was to see a downward trend in the toe temperature. There was a saying that a patient was doing well if he or she was awake, warm, and pissing.

At eight a.m., after rounds, I went with Mustafa down to the operating room. We scrubbed in. On the operating table was a little baby, covered in blue towels and ready for surgery. Mustafa made the first incision, and blood welled up from the sternum. He took a small bone saw to cut through the sternum and expose the heart. As soon as he did, the baby's heart fibrillated and stopped pumping. Mustafa quickly opened the sac of the heart, the pericardium, and started to massage the little heart, which was about the size of a hen's egg. Someone alerted Mr. Lincoln in the surgeon's waiting room. He burst through the operating room doors in his street clothes, and, cursing, pushed Mustafa aside. He asked for the defibrillating paddles and got the heart restarted almost immediately. I'd had my first important lesson—heart surgery is a matter of life and death.

Lincoln went out, scrubbed in, and came back into the OR. I stood silently at Mustafa's side for the four-hour surgery. The scrub nurse was opposite me, and to her left was Lincoln. I did not speak, and I was not spoken to. After we came off bypass, the little heart beat steadily. The baby was now pink instead of blue. Lincoln went out to the surgeon's room to have coffee, chat with the other surgeons, and dictate some notes. Mustafa changed sides, taking Lincoln's place, and I stood opposite Mustafa to help close the chest. The next baby was already being put to sleep. As soon as we had put the final sutures in, the dressings were put on and the baby was wheeled out. The next baby was wheeled in. We started again.

As we worked, we got word that the first baby had started to bleed in the intensive care unit. Sometimes when the body warms up again after bypass, small vessels that had been dry start bleeding. Possibly one of the many suture lines had come loose, or a needle hole was leaking. We finished, and the first baby was brought back in. Lincoln also came in. We reopened the incision. A small artery on the breastbone was causing the trouble. It was easily cauterized. Lincoln left, and once more Mustafa and I closed.

When we were done, it was seven p.m. It had been a long day, with nothing to eat or drink. Though I really hadn't done anything, I had learned a lot. After taking the baby back to the intensive care unit, I ran into Lincoln, who was sitting in the surgeon's room with his feet on the table. He put his tea down and gave me a careful look.

"What did you say your name was?" he said finally.

"Jamieson, sir," I stammered.

"Well, Jamieson, you didn't have a very good first day, did you?"

I wondered if my career in heart surgery had ended before it began.

Every day was an adventure, like going into the African bush with a chance of encountering almost anything. Lung surgery had been well worked out at the Brompton, which had done more of it than any other hospital in the world. The lung surgeons there were masters. But when I started, only six hundred coronary-bypass operations were done during the year in the whole of England. The senior surgeons at the Brompton had had to learn coronary surgery late in their careers. One big difference was the extremely fine suturing required in coronary surgery.

I got into a routine. Lincoln remained irritable, unpredictable, and hard to please. The days were not without mishap. Nothing was ever Lincoln's fault. There was always someone else to blame. We learned to live with it. One of the registrars told me that Lincoln had a special instrument that he kept locked away and that only he could use. "It's called the

Lincoln retrospectoscope," the registrar said. "Lincoln uses it when something has gone wrong. He looks through it like a telescope to identify the guilty party. However, it's missing an important attachment. A mirror."

I did not work directly for Paneth, but when I could, I assisted at his surgeries and covered his patients on nights and weekends. He was not like Lincoln. Tall and always expensively dressed, Paneth had a patrician air. He drove a Porsche. More interesting to me was that he had studied at the University of Minnesota under Walt Lillehei, alongside Norman Shumway and Christiaan Barnard.

Paneth was reserved outside the OR—and a supreme ruler inside it. It was not unusual for him to throw an instrument in frustration, and his nurses were sometimes reduced to tears. But his technical skills were breathtaking. I never saw a better lung surgeon. He also had his own way of working on heart valves, especially the mitral valve, which regulates blood flow between the left chambers of the heart. Most surgeons then would simply replace a bad mitral valve with an artificial one. But Paneth *repaired* the valve, using plastic-surgery methods.

CHAPTER THIRTEEN

MR. LENNOX WOULD LIKE TO KNOW WHAT THE PROBLEM IS

Three years passed. In 1974, five years after I first attended a meeting of the Transplantation Society with the money from the Rothschild prize, I went again. This time the meeting was in Jerusalem. Evelyn Rothschild made some calls on my behalf, and although I was an anonymous surgical resident, I was treated like a VIP. I was invited to lunch by the dean of Hadassah hospital and medical school, where I renewed my acquaintance with Tom Starzl. I had met Dr. Starzl—the liver-transplant pioneer—when I first worked in Ken Porter's lab. He was a giant in the field of transplantation.

I was impressed by how energetic and full of life everyone in Israel seemed to be. The country was between wars. A former Miss Israel, who was about my age, served as my escort. She was beautiful and fun. We had a marvelous time together, and I was sorry to leave.

At Christmastime in 1976, I made my last visit to Ascott. Paneth knew that I was close to Mrs. Rothschild and made sure I could get away. I think he was amused that one of the richest people in the world took such an interest in me. When I arrived Mrs. Rothschild was seriously ill. Over the holiday I think we both realized the end was coming. When I left on New Year's Eve, Yvonne hugged me. "Happy New Year," she said, "and goodbye, darling." I went back to the Brompton and threw myself into work. One day Paneth called me into his office. This was never a good thing, and I wondered what I could have done wrong.

"You'd better sit down, Jamieson," he said. "Mrs. Rothschild has died."

I was brokenhearted. Although I kept clothing and books at Ascott—it really had become my second home—I could not bear to retrieve them. Instead, I did the only thing that relieved the pain: I worked. It was now 1977. I had been a doctor for six years and finished all the requirements for general surgery. I was a fellow of the Royal College of Surgeons, Mr. Jamieson. I was appointed a senior registrar, to work mainly with Paneth.

Patients still died all the time, though nobody was keeping score back then. Today you're in trouble if you lose a patient doing heart-valve surgery. But back then surgery was often bloody, the outcome uncertain. If we did a valve and lost the patient in the OR, or later on in the night, we'd take the valve out, clean it up and sterilize it, and put it in somebody else the next day.

Paneth was always the lead surgeon on valve operations. The registrar assisted. I'd only been working for him for a few days when a complicated case appeared on the schedule. It was a young guy from Wales, only in his twenties. He needed an aortic-valve replacement. I wanted to do it. So I went to see Paneth.

"Mr. Paneth, I'd like to do this case," I said. Paneth was indignant. I might as well have asked if I could borrow the Porsche to take his daughter out.

"Look here, Jamieson, just who in the hell do you think you are?" he said.

"Sir, I think I'm the best registrar you'll ever have," I said.

Paneth stared at me. This was a make-or-break moment. I knew that I was either in or about to be fired.

"All right," he said finally.

I was in.

Paneth assisted on the operation, the first time he'd ever done that for a registrar. The operation went well. When it was finished, I went out to the waiting area to talk with the man's young wife, who had never been in London before. I was feeling like the king of the world. I told her that everything had gone perfectly and reassured her that her husband would be fine. Relieved, she went off to the pub. While she was there, the provisional Irish Republican Army detonated a bomb directly outside. When her husband woke up the next morning, I had to tell him that he was doing well but that his wife had lost a leg overnight.

After that, Paneth let me do a number of cases. And eventually he let me operate on my own. He'd be in the next room, maybe having a cup of coffee, but he was there if I needed him. I spent the year doing heart surgery as Paneth's apprentice. I rarely went home and often worked through the night and into the next day. When Paneth operated I opened and closed, looked after the patients, and dealt with the nurses and hospital staff. But when Paneth was away, I stepped into his shoes. This would not have been easy even with an experienced team backing me up. But that wasn't usually the case. The Brompton wasn't a teaching hospital. I had to learn a lot of things on my own. When I operated I was given the most junior anesthetists and scrub nurses when I really needed the most senior.

I worked with a surgeon named Silvio, whom I didn't like. He was careless and always making a joke at the wrong moment. We would do three or four cases a day, moving between ORs. I often opened or closed a case while Silvio helped Paneth. Occasionally Silvio would be allowed to close a case if it seemed simple enough. Closing is more than just sewing up the incision. You have to make sure nothing is bleeding and stop anything that is. And you have to be sure nothing has been overlooked and all surgical equipment is accounted for.

One day we operated on a private case, an English lord with lung cancer. When Paneth and I finished the surgery, Paneth moved to another room to do a heart case. Silvio went with him. Paneth sent for me ten minutes later—he didn't say why, but I could guess Silvio wasn't up to it. I swapped places with Silvio, who closed the lord's chest. When we reviewed the X-rays later that day, I saw what looked like a sponge in the lord's chest. I phoned Paneth at home.

"Where is it?" he asked. I told him it was at the base of the lungs, at the back.

"Where it always is," he said. "Well, we'll take it out in the morning."

I squared the situation with the patient and his family. They took it well. The next morning, Paneth and I operated and fished out the sponge. Silvio, standing idly at the head of the table asked, "Is that what you would call a spongioma?" He was joking that it was a type of sponge tumor. I wanted to choke him. Paneth was seething.

"No, Silvio, this is a sponge," he said coldly.

Silvio had left the sponge in, but I had been in charge. It was my responsibility. Silvio showed no remorse and declined to admit that he had done it. After we were out of the OR, Paneth pulled me aside.

"You closed the chest?" he asked. He knew I hadn't.

"Yes," I said.

"Swab count reported as correct?"

"Yes, sir."

"You're a member of the Medical Defense Council?" he said, referring to our malpractice insurance.

"Yes," I said. I realized suddenly that he was pulling my leg. Even so, I was shaken. I felt I had let Paneth down.

He thought things over for a minute.

"I don't want you to be depressed about it," he said at last. "Nobody will say you leave swabs behind."

A few days later, seeing that I was still upset, Paneth talked to me again, this time to tell me a story about Russell Brock. Lord Brock had been a legendary surgeon, the first at the Brompton to use the heart-lung machine. Paneth had been his senior registrar.

"We were going through a very bad time," Paneth recalled. "Everybody we did died, and it was demoralizing for the whole unit. One day I said to Brock, 'How do you manage, sir, all these people dying all over the place?' He said, 'Well, when I get up in the morning, I look in the mirror and I say to myself, Brock, who are you going to kill today?'

"Well, that's it. You can't be flippant about it, but you do your best and don't let it get you down. You can do no more."

But I never forgave Silvio. The last straw came when Paneth had done a coronary bypass, grafting a vein from the leg to restore blood supply to the heart. Although none could match his expertise in lung surgery, and few could match him in valve surgery, Paneth had learned coronary-artery surgery later in life. The delicate suturing was a challenge for him, and his stitches sometimes leaked. On this occasion I was with the patient in the intensive care unit after Paneth had left for the evening when the patient started to bleed. I monitored the situation for a while before deciding the bleeding wasn't going to stop on its own. We needed to go back to the operating room. Paneth was in the middle of dinner when I phoned. "You can take care of it, Jamieson, can't you?" he said. Certainly, I said.

I called in the operating room staff and the anesthetist, a young South African with whom I got on well. All was ready about a half hour later. The patient's blood pressure was now going down. I was hanging blood, trying to replace what he was losing. When the anesthetist arrived, we wheeled the patient into the elevator. The intensive care unit was on the fourth floor, the operating rooms on the first. The patient's blood pressure fell precipitously in the elevator, and the anesthetist gave him a shot of adrenaline. This made the pressure shoot up. But it also worsened his bleeding, which was really going now.

We rushed into the OR, and I opened the chest immediately. It was full of blood and blood clot. Silvio began removing the clot with a suction hose. He wasn't careful enough. Suddenly the graft was sucked into the tube and broke free from the aorta and the heart, ending up in the vacuum canister on the wall twelve feet away. I was horrified. Incredibly, Silvio thought it was funny and started laughing. I knew we needed Paneth and called him again. While he hurried to the hospital, I retrieved another segment of vein from the patient's leg. When Paneth got there, we sewed the graft back on. Of course, I again took full responsibility. It was a miracle that I wasn't fired.

Paneth must have known more than I told him, because it wasn't long until Silvio disappeared. He was replaced by an American, Steve Rubin. Rubin was an altogether different type. He was smart, decent, and a good doctor. I enjoyed working with him. Rubin had served in Vietnam. His battlefield experience came in handy one night when an elderly woman we'd operated on became confused, opened the window, and jumped out. She landed on one of the spiked railings that are so common in London and was hanging from a leg that had been impaled. Rubin rushed out and performed triage there in the street. After we got her inside, Steve went to the OR and amputated her leg.

I never went home. I slept in a room on the fourth floor, next to the intensive care unit. My life was operating, ward rounds, and more surgery. I was exhausted. I woke up one morning at six a.m. after five uninterrupted hours of sleep and felt refreshed.

One day Rubin called me to say that an old lady on whom we had operated had gone blue and motley. I must not have sounded concerned. "She has skin worse than an alligator!" Rubin said. I was still just listening. "Put it this way," Rubin finally said, "the anesthetist just intubated her without any sedation." Intubation—putting a large breathing tube down a patient's throat—is almost impossible to do on a conscious person.

When I got there, the cardiologists thought the woman had a pulmonary embolism, a blood clot in her lungs. This was serious. Paneth arrived, examined the patient carefully, listened to her chest, and said, "No, an embolus doesn't sound wheezy." Instead, Paneth ordered a shot of steroids and a bronchodilator. It was only asthma. The woman got better.

....

Paneth's busy practice included heart and lung surgery for adults and children. At least half of his patients were private, paying cases. Many came from other countries. They were treated the same as all the other patients who were done under the health service, except that Paneth always did their surgery.

Pediatric heart surgery was more risky then than it is now. One winter day we operated on a child from Saudi Arabia, a private patient. The surgery wasn't scheduled for another day or two, but the baby became critical. We couldn't find the father for permission, so the pediatrician signed off and we went into the OR early in the evening. During the surgery there was a lot of blood—way too much. The scissors must have gone through the back of the aorta, or maybe the pulmonary artery. The child died on the operating table.

I had to find the father and talk to him. He was inconsolable. A day later, we were due to operate on another Saudi baby, but the father came in the night before the surgery and took the child away.

I did my first solo open-heart case on February 1, 1977. The patient had a hole in the entrance chamber of the heart, the same defect that John Lewis repaired in Jacqueline Johnson in 1952, when she was five. Just twenty-four years later, it was now routine. Unlike Lewis, who was racing against the clock, I could put the child on bypass with the heart-lung machine and take my time. I was ready. It occurred to me that I was twenty-nine, and so was Jacqueline Johnson. The operation went smoothly.

I soon felt comfortable doing both heart and lung cases. In most ways, the heart cases were easier. In open-heart surgery, the heart-lung machine was a safety net, giving you time to fix anything that went wrong. Soon I was regularly doing cases alone, lung cases, mainly for cancer, and open-heart cases using the heart-lung machine. It was reassuring to know that Paneth was somewhere nearby, probably having a cup of coffee, in case I got into trouble.

But on one occasion, Paneth went out of town for a week, leaving me with several cases. One was a baby, a girl with a persistent ductus arteriosus. The ductus arteriosus is a short vessel that runs between the aorta and the pulmonary artery that allows the blood to bypass the lungs when you're in utero and not breathing air. After you're born, it closes. When it doesn't close on its own, surgery is usually required. On the day of the surgery, the young mother brought the child to the door of the operating room herself and insisted on talking with me before handing the baby over. I assured her all would be well. A nurse took the baby, and she was put to sleep.

I began the operation. The tissue of the ductus is friable—that is, it's thin and falls apart easily. Paneth insisted that the ductus should be cut, not tied off or clipped, as many other surgeons did. I clamped off the duct, cut it, and sewed up each end. When I removed the clamp from the aorta, it bled. I put the clamp back on and put another stitch in. When I took the clamp off, the bleeding was even worse.

I froze. Terrible thoughts flooded my brain. The agony of the Saudi father when I'd told him his baby had died. The stone silence in the OR when Kenyon's patient had bled out before our eyes. The anxious mother holding her child—*this* child—reluctant to hand her over. How could I go out and tell her I'd killed her baby?

I didn't dare put the clamp back on. Every time you clamp the vessel, it gets damaged. I put my finger on the aorta, and the bleeding stopped. Unable to move, I told a nurse to go get Mr. Lennox. Stuart Lennox was the only other senior surgeon in the operating complex. He worked with Paneth but was not nearly as good, and they didn't get on well.

The nurse came back after a minute and said, "Mr. Lennox would like to know what the problem is."

"Please tell him I'm doing a duct and it's bleeding." The nurse went out again. When she came back, she said Mr. Lennox said he would come when he could. I don't think he was doing anything so important that he couldn't interrupt it, but he made me wait with my finger in the baby's chest for at least ten minutes. Finally he barged in, pushed me to the side and looked the situation over for a second. He asked the nurse for a suture, put in a stitch, and walked out.

The bleeding was stopped.

I was furious with myself. I knew I could have done exactly the same thing—and probably better than Lennox had. But I'd let my emotions get in the way. I decided right there that I would never let it happen again. And it never did. Since that day I've done pioneering surgeries where the press was literally waiting outside at the doors of the OR and operated on famous people for whom an adverse outcome would have made international news. From that moment, I began to find operating relaxing. I realized I was in control and could take care of any difficulty as well as anybody else. Still, when Paneth got back, I felt that I'd let him down. Apparently Lennox went on at length about how he had to bail out an incompetent registrar. Paneth never said a word about it to me.

....

I saw patients that year who died with inoperable heart lesions, or diseases of the lung like cystic fibrosis. I was sure some of these people could have been treated with transplants. Lung transplantation wasn't being done yet, and there was a moratorium on heart transplantation in Britain owing to the many early failures.

Paneth worked mainly in the Brompton's Elizabeth ward. The head nurse in every ward at the Brompton went by the name of the ward, and so Sister Elizabeth was in charge there. I never knew her real name. I always spent a couple of hours going over all of the patients' charts before rounds with Paneth, to make sure I could answer his questions. Rounds were every Tuesday, with about twenty junior doctors and nurses trailing Paneth through the ward and crowding in to listen when he explained a case.

Sister Elizabeth was strict—the nurses were all terrified of her. I got on well enough with her, but one day we quarreled. She said nothing afterward. The next Tuesday came, and rounds began. I started discussing the first patient.

"You're talking about the wrong person, Mr. Jamieson," said Sister Elizabeth. I stared at the chart. She was right. It was the same at the next patient. I looked like an idiot. It finally dawned on me that Sister Elizabeth had moved all of the patients around randomly after I last left the ward. I never argued with her again.

I still worked in Ken Porter's lab over at St. Mary's when I could find time, transplanting hearts in rats. My days and nights were full. Then, in March, I learned Norman Shumway from Stanford would attend a meeting of the British Heart Society, where he was going to give a talk. Shumway was the only surgeon in the world doing heart transplants successfully. Knowing how keen I was to work on transplantation, Paneth had written to Shumway to ask if he would take me at Stanford for a year. Now I would have a chance to meet him.

Shumway did not usually take on outsiders. But he had previously made an exception for someone Paneth recommended. I hoped he'd make another for me. Shortly ahead of the meeting, Shumway sent a message saying his daughter had been in a car accident and he couldn't come. He sent his number two, Ed Stinson, in his place. Stinson's talk was sensational. Shumway's group had done some of the first heart transplants in animals in the late 1950s, when everyone said it was impossible. Over the next decade, they had resolved most of the problems involved in transplanting a human heart. After the initial burst of transplant activity following Christiaan Barnard's first, many surgeons abandoned the operation. Shumway carried on. Now he was doing more than half of all the heart transplants in the world.

In May, Shumway wrote to Paneth saying that he would take me for a year. But I would have to pay my own way. I wondered how much I needed to live on in California. Shumway said his residents at my level earned about $20,000 a year. I doubted I could find that much. I applied for a grant from the British Heart Foundation and started the process of getting a visa for America. It was a busy time. In my first six months working with Paneth, we did 327 cases together, 166 on the heart-lung machine. I did eighty-three on my own, including twenty-two on the heart-lung machine.

In July, everything changed. I rotated off Paneth's service and went to work for Stuart Lennox. I still covered for Paneth at nights and on weekends, but Lennox became my primary boss. We had fewer cases. Lennox often changed his technique. Every time he went to a meeting or visited another center, usually overseas, he would come back with a different way of doing things. I thought this was a mistake, that it was important to stick to a reliable method that worked well in your hands. Plus, Lennox was sloppy when he tried something new; I never saw him following the recommended procedure precisely. When he got excited in the operating room, which was often, he would scream, "Pass me my whatsit." With no idea what he was talking about, the nurse would hand him an instrument that seemed right. "No," he would shout, "Give me the other one." Sometimes it was difficult not to laugh. Fortunately, as I got to know him, Lennox turned out to be a friendly sort, less intimidating, certainly, than Paneth.

As I was less busy than I had been with Paneth, I asked Lennox if I could put together a team to try heart transplants in dogs. He was hesitant but finally relented. I got a small grant and permission from the Home Office to work on dogs—something that had become a sensitive topic with the emerging animal-rights movement. The work went well. At night the team went home and I dozed on the floor of the laboratory next to the dogs, so that I could check on them from time to time.

Around this time, Christiaan Barnard was in the news again. He had transplanted a baboon heart into a person with heart failure. I was amazed that even someone as reckless at Barnard would not know that the baboon heart would be quickly rejected because of the cross-species reaction. The patient did not survive.

In October that year, Denton Cooley, the renowned Texas heart surgeon, came to visit. He was speaking to the British Heart Society, and I was assigned to meet him at the airport. He was unmistakable when he stepped off the plane, accompanied by his wife, Louise. He was tall, self-assured, and spoke with a Texas twang. I liked him right off.

Cooley did an operation while he was with us, a coronary bypass. I assisted. At first he didn't seem to be fast, though that was his reputation. But he was fast. There were no wasted moves. He never did anything twice and never checked what he did because he knew it was right. Every move was deliberate and perfect. He was calm and polite, and this mood took over the OR. It was pleasure to watch him at work, and the surgery was over before I knew it.

When I drove Cooley and his wife back to the airport, he told me that it was essential for me go to the United States to see different ways of doing things. I did not know then that our paths would cross many times, and that we would become friends. Twenty years after I dropped him off at the airport, we attended an event together. It was Cooley's job to introduce me. When he did, he kept it short. "Stuart Jamieson is here with us tonight. He's the second best heart surgeon in the world."

In December, the British Heart Foundation gave me a scholarship of $12,000, a little more than half the amount Shumway said that his fellows were paid. I figured I could manage somehow.

Paneth asked me to come to his office late one afternoon. When I went in, he told me to close the door and take a seat. He said that they would appoint someone temporarily to keep my senior registrar job open while I was at Stanford. He said a number of people at the Brompton thought I would make a good replacement for one of the senior surgeons who was retiring soon. I was flattered. The idea that I could become a consultant when I'd just turned thirty was exhilarating.

My year at the Brompton came to an end. I had been in the OR for more than seven hundred cases, about a third of which I had done myself. I had not taken a single day off. And it had been wonderful.

CHAPTER FOURTEEN
THE BEATING HEART

Norman Shumway was in the observation balcony at the University of Minnesota when John Lewis did the first open-heart surgery in 1952. He had done his PhD under Lewis on the effects of hypothermia on the heart. Now that the heart-lung machine could keep the body alive and perfused with blood for two or three hours, cooling the whole body during heart surgery was not necessary. When Shumway moved to Stanford, he performed experiments in dogs to see if cooling only the heart would protect it without a blood supply for an hour or so while he worked on it. With a dog on the heart-lung machine, Shumway removed the heart and then sewed it back in again. This proved to be difficult, because there wasn't much left to sew it to. So next they transplanted a heart from another dog, leaving connective tissues from the original organ in place to which the new heart could be attached. This led to the early transplant work in the Stanford laboratories. The technique of leaving remnants of the native heart behind to provide a rim of tissue to which the transplant could be sewn became known as the Shumway technique. It would eventually be used in human transplants.

In fact, working on dogs was excellent preparation for working on humans. Dog tissues are more friable and likely to come apart after suturing than human tissues are. If you can operate on a dog, you can operate on a human.

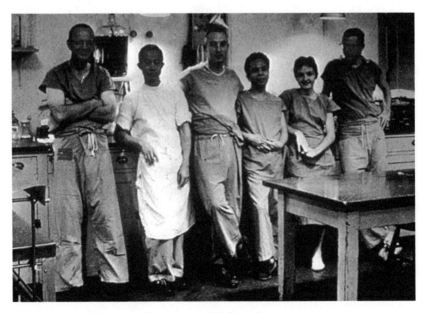

Norman Shumway with his laboratory team.
On the left is Ray Stofer, who ran the heart-lung machine.
On the right is Richard Lower, who later started a heart
transplant program in Richmond, Virginia.

Photograph courtesy of Dr. Shumway

By 1959, Shumway believed their short-term results with transplants in dogs were good enough to present to the American College of Surgeons' meeting that year in Atlantic City. Dick Lower, a member of Shumway's team, delivered the paper while Shumway listened. Shumway later said that there was so little interest in their work that Lower had spoken to an audience consisting of "the chairman of the session, myself, and the projectionist."

But the Shumway group forged ahead, working out the basic principles of heart transplantation. Would a transplanted heart beat in a normal rhythm? Yes, they found. Would it support circulation in the recipient? The answer to that was also yes. And they discovered that if the donor heart was immersed in a cold saline solution, it could be transported to the recipient and still function properly. That left only one problem, but it was the big one: how to prevent rejection of the transplanted heart. Untreated, the animals rejected their hearts in a period of five to ten days.

Shumway's team tried an array of immunosuppressive drugs, searching for one, or a combination, that would depress the body's natural defensive response but not so much that the organ recipient was overwhelmed by infection. Here their progress was more halting. They tried azathiaprine—Imuran—which had been under investigation as an immune suppressant since the late 1950s. Various steroids were tested. So were radiation and antithymocyte globulin—ATG—a serum created in rabbits that carries antibodies against rejection cells. This was painstaking work, but by the early 1960s they'd had some success. One dog, Ralphie, had lived more than a year after transplantation.

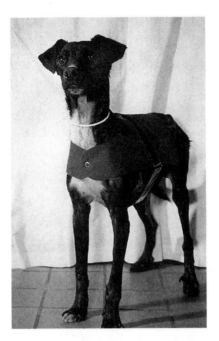

Ralphie. The first living thing to have survived a year after a heart transplant. 1964.

Photograph courtesy of Dr. Shumway

Some of Shumway's research would have troubled animal rights groups and medical ethicists had word got around. In 1966, Dick Lower transplanted a heart from a human cadaver into a chimpanzee. The heart functioned for a few hours, at which point Lower euthanized the chimp and terminated the experiment. Nothing was said about this, but it was the first heart transplant using a human donor.

<hr />

By 1967, at least four surgeons in the US were poised to transplant a human heart: Norman Shumway at Stanford; Dick Lower, now working in Virginia; James Hardy at the University of Mississippi; and Adrian Kantrowitz in New York. The shocking news that Christiaan Barnard in South Africa had beaten them all to it had to be discouraging. Dr. Shumway, who as I was soon to learn was unfailingly kind and generous, wrote to Barnard to congratulate him. Had Shumway been able to find a donor a few months earlier, history would have been different.

On January 6, 1968, Shumway finally had his donor, and the world's fourth heart transplant took place at Stanford. The recipient was a fifty-four-year-old steel worker, Mike Kasperak, from East Palo Alto. In retrospect, he was a bad candidate for a transplant. Besides being terminally ill, he also had kidney failure and generalized atherosclerosis.

Ed Stinson, Shumway's chief resident, assisted. He later said the operation had been "awe-inspiring." It was also a moment when the team reflected on the moral and legal implications of what they were doing. At the time there was no brain-death standard in California. A person was declared dead when their heart stopped beating.

"After we removed the recipient's heart," Stinson said, "we stared at the empty pericardial cavity for a good half minute and wondered what we'd actually done." Stinson asked Shumway if it was legal. Shumway shrugged and continued working. "I'm not sure," he said. "Time will tell." When the new heart was in place, nothing happened at first. Then it started to beat a little. Pretty soon the heartbeat became strong. Mike Kasperak lived for fourteen days before he died of kidney failure and sepsis.

Shumway hated publicity, but the transplant operation was big news. Reporters climbed the walls of the hospital to try to get a peek into the operating room. And around the world in the coming months, surgeons began doing heart transplants every few days. Sadly, only Shumway and Lower—who had now moved on to Virginia—understood enough about rejection, both the process itself and also how to diagnose it, a critical consideration in trying to balance immune suppression. Eight of Shumway's first heart transplant patients lived for more than a year after their surgery. Dick Lower's first patient died after a week. But his second would survive for more than six years.

Inevitably, though, heart transplants produced dismal results in most of the cardiac centers that tried them. Denton Cooley in Houston did more heart transplants than anyone in the world that year—twenty. None of the recipients survived past eighteen months. In all, 80 percent of the world's transplant recipients died within a year. It was true that *all* of these patients would have died without transplant surgery, but critics argued that the expense and the emotional toll of extending life by a few days or months was not worth it.

In 1971, the Stanford group published their results with twenty-six human heart transplant patients. Nearly half had survived for six months, and one in four was alive two years after surgery. Nobody else was even close. The key to survival of the patients had been the diagnosis and treatment of early rejection.

Philip Caves, a visiting fellow from the Brompton whom Paneth had sent to Shumway, introduced another major advance at Stanford in 1973 that furthered their ability to detect early rejection. It was a method to biopsy the heart. A long forceps was introduced through a neck vein and passed down into the heart, where small tissue samples could be taken. For the first time, it was possible to directly observe the rejection process. This was a tremendous development. By 1974, the Stanford group had performed fifty-nine human heart transplants, with survival rates of 43 percent at one year, 40 percent at two years, and 26 percent at three years. These numbers improved steadily over the next few years. Meanwhile, in Cape Town, Christiaan Barnard's team did only ten heart transplants between 1967 and 1973. Barnard spent more time giving lectures and jet-setting than he did operating, in love with his fame and, as he later confessed, with the endless succession of young women eager to sleep with him at every stop.

In the end, the race had been won not by the swift, but by the careful. While he hadn't been the first, Shumway was soon regarded everywhere as the father of heart transplantation. Stanford was where I had to go.

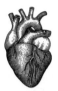

PART THREE

AMERICA

CHAPTER FIFTEEN

NOBODY THREW INSTRUMENTS ON THE FLOOR

I went to America at the beginning of 1978, leaving behind my sports car, my apartment, and my life in London—not to mention an ascendant career at the Brompton. Not long before I left, I was interviewed for a multi-institutional job as senior surgical registrar at the Brompton, the National Heart Hospital, and the London Chest Hospital. Competition for the job was intense. Of the many applicants, I was the youngest. At the end of the interview, after discussing my experience, I was asked about the rest of my life.

"What are your hobbies?"

I said I had none.

"Well, what do you do in your spare time?"

Again, I said I had none.

"Well, then, how do you relax?"

I said I relaxed in the OR.

I was offered the job.

But America beckoned. The future of heart transplantation was being born at Stanford, and I desperately wanted to be part of it. I took a deep breath and turned my back on what many heart surgeons would have considered the chance of a lifetime.

California reminded me of Rhodesia. After a decade in England, it was like coming home. The smells, the weather, the flowers were all familiar in a way the concrete gloom of London never could be. Shumway had sent a car to meet me at the airport, something that I was to learn later he rarely did. The driver, holding a sign with "Dr. Jamieson" on it, was waiting for me in baggage claim. We drove down Highway 101, and he dropped me at the Riviera Motor Lodge in Palo Alto. It had been a long trip, but I quickly showered and was soon hurrying across an immense parking lot—the hotel was next to a shopping center, something I'd had little experience with—in search of the Stanford hospital. When I got there and asked for directions to Shumway's office, I was surprised that nobody seemed to know who he was.

I found Shumway in a nondescript wing of the hospital. I was excited to meet the hero of heart transplantation, who at fifty-four was in the prime of his career. He was dressed in scrubs. Shumway led me into his modest, uncarpeted office. There was a small desk and one chair in it. The room itself was barely big enough for the furniture. Shumway asked me to sit down and perched himself on the edge of the desk. As I would see in the coming months, Shumway never made a show of being an internationally acclaimed surgeon. He seemed to be content that nobody at Stanford paid him much attention. This only elevated my opinion of him.

We talked for a half hour. Shumway asked about Paneth, the Brompton, and my expectations for the coming year at

Stanford. I told him I wanted to do clinical work, and that I was mainly interested in heart surgery and transplantation.

"You'd better go see Patrick Rooney," he said.

Rooney was Shumway's chief resident. He was tall, wore glasses and had a broken nose. He'd been in the navy after medical school. After that he'd done a residency in cardiology before starting in general surgery and then cardiothoracic surgery at Stanford. He was older than most of the senior residents, always composed, and a great clinician. When Rooney wasn't in the OR, he was always smoking a cigarette, carrying it in his left hand and holding a can of Coca-Cola in his right. I was delighted that he seemed to like me.

My fellowship stipend wasn't enough to live on and cover my obligations in London. Somehow I'd have to stretch my meager resources. It began to sink in that I was starting over in more ways than one. Working with Paneth, I'd been doing heart surgery on my own. At Stanford I was the most junior person in Shumway's group, and as far as they were concerned, a nobody. I would have to prove myself all over again.

I was also a stranger in a new country. Having rarely left the hospital in London for the past several years, I was ignorant about many things that are a routine part of daily life for people who don't work nonstop. As soon as I could, I bought a secondhand bicycle to get around on. I read something about how you were supposed to have a license for a bike. So I set off to find one. After making some inquiries and getting a lot of funny looks, I was told that I might get a license at the fire station. The firemen were amused when I explained what I wanted. But they dug around and managed to find a bicycle license, which I purchased and dutifully attached to the bike, taking care to follow the instructions about affixing it to the wheel hub. I think it was the only bicycle license they had ever issued. And I've never come across anyone else who had one. I soon learned that Britain is less keen about rules than America is, but in Britain you don't break those rules. America is awash in regulations, but many are ignored or winked at.

I found an apartment in East Palo Alto, the wrong side of the tracks. It was a poor area and generally regarded as unsafe at that time. The apartment was just one room on the ground floor of a flimsy-looking complex. I didn't think too much about it because I knew I'd stay at the hospital most of the time. When I did go home, I rode my bike each way, usually in the dark. It was a rainy year, and I'd get home or to work soaked through. In London I'd taken to wearing cowboy boots, and now found that everybody in Shumway's group did, but these would fill with water on the way, increasing my misery. I'd expected California to be hot and dry.

One night as I was riding home, I saw a garbage can by the curb that had a coat hanging out of it. I stopped. The coat was old and worn but serviceable. I put it on and went home. I kept it for many years, long after I could afford a new one, to remind me of the days when I couldn't.

I hadn't been at Stanford long when I arrived home one night to find my apartment door open. The place had been ransacked. As far I could tell, nothing was gone. I mentioned the incident to Shumway, telling him it was humiliating that at age thirty, having worked hard all my life, I had accumulated nothing worth stealing in even the poorest part of town. He laughed and said the burglars must have figured I was one of them and let me keep my things. On another night, I came home in the dark to find a bullet hole in the window. I dug the spent bullet out of the wall.

I learned how dangerous East Palo Alto was when we had a young boy from Belgium in for a heart transplant. His father had come with him, and while the boy was recovering after surgery, the father visited a bar in my neighborhood. He was accosted by a man with a gun demanding money. Things like that didn't happen in Belgium, and the father refused to turn over his wallet. The gunman shot him in the pelvis and took his money. The father was brought in to the emergency room at Stanford. His femoral artery and femoral vein were lacerated, and he was bleeding badly. We operated and saved his life. Unfortunately, his son had severe rejection and never left the hospital.

For the first six months of 1978, I worked as a junior resident. This turned out to consist almost entirely of looking after post-operative patients. On a good day, I might be allowed into the operating room to harvest a vein for a coronary bypass operation. Shumway's group had a saying that until you had taken a hundred miles of vein, you weren't allowed to do heart operations.

The other junior resident was Ronald Ponn. Ponn was from Boston and came from money. He lived in a big house on a hill with his second wife. Ponn talked while holding a cigarette between his teeth. We spent most of our time in the intensive care unit that was reserved for Shumway's heart-surgery patients. The nurses on the unit were assertive, as they had to be, and functioned like junior doctors. They knew a lot, and you were well advised to listen to them.

Shumway seemed always to know everything that went on in the hospital, every detail about the patients, about the staff, about the nurses, even the gossip. He managed this by being on good terms with the nurses, who called him Uncle Norm. Nothing happened that the nurses didn't know about, and they confided in Shumway, who never let anyone think he was their superior.

Shumway's lieutenants were Ed Stinson, whom I'd heard speak in London, and Phil Oyer. They were close friends and unconventional. Ed chain-smoked. Phil chewed tobacco. They always wore cowboy boots. Once a year they would go on a horseback cattle roundup together, driving a herd of cattle from its summer to winter pastures. Both of them loved guns. Ed was skinny as a rake, and we used to say that even his tapeworm had a tapeworm. One weekend he shot himself in the leg while practicing his quick draw. He was brought to the emergency room at Stanford. The wound wasn't serious—he'd managed to miss everything important. The emergency room doctor called Shumway at home and said, "Ed Stinson has just shot himself."

"Well, I knew things were bad," Shumway said drily, "but surely not that bad."

Stinson and Oyer were unflappable in the operating room. Ed always wore a red bandanna tied around his head instead of the standard cap. There were two ORs on the cardiac unit. Shumway was in room 13, Ed and Phil in room 12. Ed and Phil's service was called *l'otro*, "the other," service. Shumway was before his time in believing that a general surgery board certification was unnecessary for a cardiovascular surgeon. Both Ed and Phil had skipped years of general surgical training to gain extra time in cardiac surgery. They were among the best I'd ever seen. Neither had taken the general surgery boards, which meant they weren't certified in cardiac surgery, either, because you needed general surgery boards in order to take the cardiac surgery boards. It took years for others to see it Shumway's way. Today, both in Europe and the United States, surgeons going into cardiac work spend less time in general surgery, which makes sense.

Oyer was experimenting with a left ventricular-assist device. This was an implantable electrical pump that took blood from the left ventricle, the main pumping chamber of the heart, and pumped it into the aorta, the main artery to the body. The idea was to develop an assist device that could buy time for a patient waiting for a transplant. Such a device could always be on hand and would require no immunosuppression. Oyer spent every Thursday on this project, putting the pump into calves, checking the feasibility of the surgery, and studying the hemodynamics—that is, how effectively the pump could take over the circulation. Phil's research led to the first practical artificial heart-support device.

My first six months at Stanford were not a happy time. I was cold and miserable. I found the work tedious and uninspiring. One morning, on my way in at around five a.m. in a downpour, the chain came off my bicycle and I crashed into a ditch, badly scraping both arms and one leg. I lay next to the broken bicycle in the dark, bleeding and in pain, wondering how I could have done this to myself. My career was going in reverse. I thought about being back at the Brompton, doing heart surgery on my own every day, driving around London in the Triumph. But I realized that going back would be admitting defeat. I had to stick it out.

....

Ron Ponn and I alternated every other night on call, sleeping in a bed in the intensive care unit. But I rarely went home on my off nights. There wasn't much point in riding back to my crummy apartment only to get up again a few hours later to shower and ride back to Stanford, still in the dark. It was easier to stay at the hospital, where it was warm, food was available in the cafeteria downstairs, and I could keep an eye on the patients. When Shumway had performed a particularly challenging operation on a child who was unstable afterward, I napped in a chair at the foot of the bed even if Ron was on call that night. He would be busy enough, as the rest of the beds in the intensive care unit were usually full.

Not everything was bleak. I learned new techniques and experienced a different atmosphere in the OR. At the Brompton there was often tension in the air. Senior surgeons thought nothing of exploding angrily at someone in the middle of an operation. At Stanford, it was relaxed. There were no raised voices. Nobody threw instruments on the floor or looked for somebody to blame when a mistake happened. Operating was calm and fun. Shumway had a sense of humor. In difficult moments, he would relax everybody by telling a joke while the problem got fixed.

Shumway was not particularly fast in the operating room, but his judgment was impeccable. He always knew just what to do, and how to do just enough and no more. Paneth may have been technically better, but it was Shumway's judgment that set him apart. I've long since realized that this, more than anything else, is the hallmark of a great surgeon.

There are a few people who become surgeons who are complete naturals. They're born with a knife in their hands. And then there are the majority, who work hard and become competent. And there are a few who should not be allowed inside an OR. But technical skill doesn't count for much if you lack judgment.

Say you have an eighty-five-year-old woman who needs an aortic valve replaced. Many of the heart surgery patients we see have multiple problems. So maybe in addition to the aortic valve there's a partial blockage in a coronary artery, the aorta has a minor aneurysm, and the mitral valve leaks a little, too. Your job is to give this patient another few years of life—not to fix everything that's wrong with her. You have to know when to stop. In a case like this, you do the aortic valve and close her up. A surgeon without good judgment will do more than is necessary, repair all of it, and then be surprised when the patient never comes off the heart-lung machine. When you worked with Shumway, you learned that in heart surgery, less can be more.

I never missed an opportunity to be involved in a transplant case. I went out on the donor runs, flying to remote hospitals to retrieve a heart. These were still early days, and nobody else in California was transplanting hearts. That meant that we had no competition for donors. We took an operating room nurse, a technician, and a medical student with us. We'd get on a plane, often at night, wearing scrubs. Time was critical, especially on the return. The longer the heart was out of the body, the greater the risk to the recipient. On one donor run, we flew to a hospital about five hundred miles from Stanford. After taking out the heart and putting it on ice, we rushed back to the small airfield in the early hours of the morning and took off into the dark. Well into the return flight, we realized we had left the scrub nurse behind. She had gone to the bathroom in the airport, and we had departed in our customary haste without noticing she wasn't onboard. We didn't have the time to go back. The nurse reappeared at Stanford three days later, still in her scrubs, and unhappy. She had not taken any money with her and must have had a rough trip back. There were no cell phones then, of course. We never got the full story, because it was several weeks before she would speak to us.

....

Heart transplantation was moving ahead slowly everywhere but at Stanford, and was halted altogether in England. I decided to review the results of the Stanford program and write them up. The paper, "Cardiac Transplantation in 150 Patients at Stanford University," reviewed all the transplants that had been carried out at Stanford between January 1968 and August 1978. This was a majority of all the heart transplants done throughout the world to that point. I submitted it to the *British Medical Journal*, which published it in January of 1979, along with an editorial noting that Stanford's one-year survival rate had now reached 70 percent, comparable to the success rate for kidney transplants. The journal's editors also pointed to the "massive research" effort at Stanford that explained our success. If heart transplants were to be restarted in England, they wrote, it should be in a cardiac center that followed the Stanford model.

As I later learned, one person in England who read the article with interest was a surgeon named Terence English. He's now Sir Terence, and a close friend. English had done heart surgery at the Brompton before I went there and had also visited Stanford to study our transplant procedures. He thought it was time for England to get back in the game. The National Health Service had refused to allow heart transplants for a decade, but English had a private patient and private money to go ahead with one. Then, just one day after my journal article appeared, and probably because of it, English got a call from Addenbrooke's Hospital in Cambridge with a donor.

English knew that any attempt to break the moratorium would attract attention, and so it had to be a success. His patient was a redo—someone who had already had heart surgery. That's not uncommon. But it makes it difficult to open the chest because of all the scar tissue. Often, the heart is stuck to the sternum. So if you just saw through the sternum like we usually do, you risk cutting a hole in the heart before you can get the patient on the heart-lung machine.

English wanted to ensure that the donor heart was good, so he went to collect it while his senior registrar opened up the recipient. The patient arrested. They did CPR and managed to resuscitate him but had no idea if he was brain-dead. The registrar phoned English and asked what to do. I've often wondered what I would have done. What English decided was that the transplant was this patient's only chance at life and they were going to go ahead.

The man never woke up, and they pulled the plug ten days later.

The press coverage was brutal. English never told anybody what happened, never made an excuse. Instead, he did another one. And this one worked. And then he did another and another. Heart transplantation in England was back.

I've always thought that if something happened to me, if I needed heart surgery, I'd want a surgeon like English. Someone who put the patient ahead of himself.

I'd completed six months on the clinical service. Shumway suggested I spend some time in the lab. The animal laboratory was on the same floor as the offices and the outpatient department. It was cramped, about eight paces wide and perhaps twenty paces long. Windows on one side opened out to the quadrangle. This was the room in which Shumway and Lower and their technicians had figured out how to make human heart transplants possible, mostly through their work in dogs.

My coworker in the lab was Nelson Burton, who was also a cardiac surgical resident. We had to store all of the lab equipment in the room overnight, so the first thing we did every day at six a.m. was move things into the corridor so we had space to work. There were two operating tables and an old heart-lung machine that had been salvaged from the OR after it was no longer used on patients. The machine had an early type of oxygenator that only worked for short periods. It was heavy and took a long time to clean after a procedure. Sometimes we'd spend the entire day cleaning and sterilizing equipment. But everything was reusable, so it was a cheap setup for experimentation.

I continued to investigate why atherosclerosis occurred in blood vessels after heart transplantation. I worked in rats, as I had done at St. Mary's—until I managed to land a grant from a drug company to buy monkeys. They were expensive and harder to care for than rats, but using primates was important. It was the best way to be sure that what we were doing in the laboratory would be applicable to humans. After more than two decades of research in dogs, monkeys arrived at the Stanford lab in July 1978.

Shumway's newest faculty member, Bruce Reitz, was in charge of the lab. He had finished his chief resident year in 1976 and subsequently done two additional years of general surgery to become board certified. Since Bruce was on the full-time faculty and had regular clinical duties, Burton and I did the day-to-day work. We had two technicians, Jesse and Grant, who were adept at putting in intravenous lines, giving anesthesia, and putting the animals on ventilators. They were excellent scrub nurses, too. It was a good team.

When we started the work in monkeys, I thought that we should be able to cut a donor heart out in such a way that we could replace it—swapping hearts between two monkeys. This meant we didn't have to sacrifice the donor monkey, and would have two subjects to study in one experiment. The problem with that was that we only had one heart-lung machine. We decided to see if we could do a heart swap using only hypothermia, the technique that Lewis had used in Jacqueline Johnson twenty-five years earlier.

The monkeys were anesthetized, placed on ventilators, and then laid in blue plastic infant bathtubs. We packed them in ice and monitored their temperatures and the EKGs. As they gradually cooled, the heart rate slowed. We found that if they were adequately anesthetized and the cooling was carried out slowly, they could be cooled to approximately 26 degrees Celsius before the heart fibrillated. At that point we took them out of the baths, put them on the operating tables, and opened them up. Burton operated on one monkey, and I did the other. We switched hearts. When the new hearts had been sewn into place, we warmed the monkeys up by pouring warm saline into their chests and placing them on heating blankets while doing cardiac massage. Soon the new hearts began to beat. We were able to do the operations in less than an hour. The monkeys recovered normally.

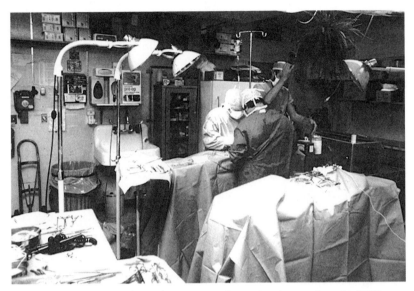

In the laboratory doing heart transplantation in monkeys in 1978. Nelson Burton (left) is being assisted by Jesse Gutierrez. Grant Hoyt is giving anesthesia. I am taking the picture, about to transplant the monkey on the right.

Charlie Bieber, a pathologist and immunologist who worked for Shumway in another laboratory next door, made the antithymocyte globulin (ATG) that we used in the transplant patients. Antibodies and lymphocytes are made in the bone marrow and thymus, a gland in the front of the neck. The gland is large in babies and slowly disappears with age. Whenever we operated on babies, we had to remove most of the thymus to gain access to the heart. We called Charlie to the operating room, where he would take the gland back to the lab, grind it up, and inject it into rabbits. After about ten days, the rabbits had made antibodies to the human lymphocytes—proteins that would in essence reject the body's own rejection response. The rabbits' blood would be removed, the red cells taken out, and the remaining serum was

ATG. It was injected into the thigh muscles of our heart transplant patients. This was excruciating because of the inflammatory reaction it caused, and the patients would hobble about for weeks. But it worked. The rabbit antibodies attacked the human cells that were trying to reject the transplanted heart. This close collaboration between the lab and the clinical practice was what enabled Stanford to perform more heart transplants than the rest of the world combined.

Although heart transplantation can extend a life by years or even decades, the patient is trading a lethal condition for a chronic one, because they have to take drugs to suppress their immune system for as long as they live. These drugs have side effects and also inhibit the body's ability to fend off infections. As good as the current immunosuppression treatment was, we knew it had to get better.

By October 1978, Nelson and I had perfected our technique of heart transplantation in monkeys using hypothermia. Almost all the animals survived. We were testing immunosuppressive regimens to stop rejection and improve survival. That month, Charlie Bieber showed me a copy of an article in the journal *Immunology*, describing a new immunosuppressive drug. Jean Borel, the author, worked for a drug company called Sandoz in Switzerland. The scientists there had been analyzing samples of earth from various places to see if they could come up with useful new antibiotics. Borel, looking at a sample from a highland plateau in Norway, found a fungus with a new structure, from which he extracted a chemical they called cyclosporin A. Later on it would be called simply cyclosporin. It was a white powder. Its antibiotic properties turned out to be nonexistent—in fact, it had the opposite effect. It inhibited the immune response. I was intrigued and talked with Charlie about whether cyclosporin might be useful in transplant patients. A group in England working mainly on liver and kidney transplants began testing cyclosporin and by the end of the year had promising results that were published in the *Lancet*, a well-known British medical journal. They'd overcome a challenge in using cyclosporin: it doesn't dissolve in water. This made it hard to work with in the lab, as it is difficult to make animals swallow a precise dose of a powder. But a young Greek researcher named Alkis Kostakis, who was visiting in England, had discovered that cyclosporin is fat soluble. You can dissolve it in olive oil.

Though Kostakis's name has been lost to history, he was responsible for a major step forward in heart transplantation. After reading the *Lancet* article, Charlie and I knew we had to get our hands on some cyclosporin. I wrote to Borel. He offered to give us a sample if someone would come to Switzerland to get it.

Phil Oyer was going to Europe toward the end of 1978. He came back with about a pound of cyclosporin in a large brown bottle, probably the first sample of cyclosporin to enter the United States. Phil kept the bottle in a drawer in his desk in his office. We had to ask him for some whenever we needed it in the laboratory. We dissolved the cyclosporin in olive oil and gave it to the animals that had had heart transplants. We started with rats, which could take the drug orally.

The results were immediately clear. Cyclosporin worked better than any other immunosuppressive drug, or any of the combinations of drugs, I had tested. I wrote up the findings of our experiments and submitted the paper to be presented at the American College of Surgeons meeting. It was accepted, and I gave the paper at the annual meeting in Chicago the next year. The proceedings of the meeting were published in a journal called *Surgical Forum* in 1979. That paper and one from Boston studying lymphocytes were the first two reports of the use of cyclosporin in the American literature.

We lost no time in studying cyclosporin in our monkeys. Monkeys had to take the drug by injection. Again, the results were impressive. Cyclosporin was more effective than anything we had tried before. The monkeys lived and seemed normal. I wrote up these results, which were published in the *Lancet*. This was the first report of cyclosporin used in heart transplants in primates.

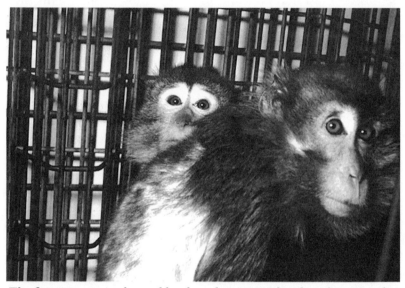

The first primates in the world to have been treated with cyclosporin after heart transplantation. The monkey on the left gave his heart to the monkey on the right, and vice-versa.

I felt that years of hard work, going back to my days as a student in Ken Porter's lab at St. Mary's, had paid off. What was most exciting about cyclosporin was that it did not impede the healing of tissues the way other drugs—especially steroids—did.

At the same time, clinical work continued to advance. Shumway was keen on revisiting the possibility of lung transplantation, which had been a clinical failure. The first lung transplant was done in 1963 by James Hardy in Mississippi. By 1978, my first year at Stanford, a total of thirty-eight lung transplants had been attempted in the world, with no long-term success. Only nine of the thirty-eight patients had lived for more than two weeks, and only one patient had been discharged alive from the hospital. He died within the year.

The main challenge in lung transplantation is that the airway does not have a rich blood supply, which is vital for healing. Most patients had died because the airway sutures broke down. Immunosuppressive drugs also interfered with the cell division that is essential to healing. Experimental work on lung transplantation in dogs had not been helpful because dogs have a different breathing mechanism from primates. After lung transplantation, dogs try to keep breathing in without exhaling. None survived for long. One glimmer of hope was an experiment in which Shumway and Dick Lower had transplanted the heart and both lungs in dogs. One of them survived briefly, and the procedure was written up in the journal *Surgery* in 1961.

That result had helped to convince Shumway that lung transplants by themselves would not work. He reasoned that if lung transplants failed because the sutures keeping the airway together didn't hold, then a better approach was to, as he put it, "Do a transplant of the whole thing—the heart and lungs attached, the heart-and-lung block." And because diseased hearts and lungs tend to co-occur in patients, being able to fix both at the same time made sense.

This approach would have two advantages. The heart has collateral arteries that also supply the airway where the suture line would be. Doing a heart-and-lung transplant would preserve much of the blood supply to the airway, which would help healing and prevent the breakdown of the suture line. In addition, the trachea, the main airway supplying both lungs, has a better blood supply than the bronchi, the smaller airways that branch off the trachea, which you had to sew together when you did a single-lung transplant. A side benefit was that rejection of the heart, which we had become good at monitoring, would signal rejection in the lungs as well.

Work on heart-and-lung transplants in the Stanford lab commenced at the end of 1978, just as I was due to return to the Brompton. Shumway approached me in the corridor one day. He never sent for anybody. He always came to find you. He wanted to know what I was doing the next year. I told him I was going back to London. He asked me what I would be doing there, and I told him I would be senior registrar at the Brompton and National Heart Hospitals—a position most people would have regarded as vastly beyond my junior status at Stanford.

"Why don't you stay another year?" Shumway asked.

I told him that I would love to.

When I phoned Paneth, he said that they could get along without me. He would appoint someone to take my place for another year and said he would ask the British Heart Foundation to extend my grant for a year. They did.

The next twelve months were exciting. Bruce Reitz took the lead on heart-and-lung transplants in the monkeys, using our hypothermia method. At first we simply removed the heart and lungs and then put them back in. We found that monkeys did not experience the same breathing problems as dogs. And there was no problem with the sutures where we had connected the airways. The airways healed well in all the monkeys with a simple suture line of polypropylene, a type of nylon. We used the nylon sutures instead of the usual absorbable sutures so they could stay in for a long time under immunosuppression. The monkeys recovered well and breathed normally. These results seemed to bode well for heart-lung transplantation in humans.

In the beginning, we used no immunosuppression to see whether the heart or the lungs would reject first. I was in the lab one Saturday night and noticed that our first monkey was having breathing difficulties. This was probably the first observation of lung rejection in a primate. I called Bruce at home, and he came in. The breathing got worse over the next few hours. This proved to be a pattern. Lung rejection was manifested by shortness of breath and came before rejection of the heart. This suggested that maybe heart rejections wouldn't be an early warning for lung rejection after all.

When we then treated the animals with cyclosporin, they did well. But cyclosporin was not a magic bullet. It had to be combined with other drugs to get the best results. We tried cyclosporin in combination with the drugs we were using in humans—Imuran, steroids, and ATG—and got long-term survivors. We called the first monkey to live for months after surgery Mom, because one of my coworkers said she looked like his mother-in-law. Mom was a milestone. We were convinced that successful heart-and-lung transplants in humans were just a matter of time.

We continued to refine the immunosuppression regimen in early 1979. Some of the monkeys developed lymphomas, a type of cancer. This indicated that their immune systems were being suppressed too much. We deleted steroids from our drug cocktail and also cut back on ATG. This worked better. I was now doing what I had always wanted to do and felt, finally, that I was playing an important part in advancing the science of organ transplantation.

At the end of a year in the lab, Shumway approached me again.

"What are you going to do next year?" he asked casually.

I told him I was going back to be senior registrar at the Brompton and National Chest Hospitals.

"Why don't you stay another year?" he said.

I called Paneth, who was not happy. But he said he would support me in whatever I wanted to do. He arranged for my financial support from the British Heart Foundation to continue. In July 1979, I became Shumway's chief resident, running his service. I was also the chief resident in charge of the heart transplant program. Everything I'd given up to come to Stanford had been regained—and then some.

CHAPTER SIXTEEN
BLOOD AND AIR

At Stanford, the chief resident did all the surgery but was always accompanied by a senior surgeon, which was different from my experience in England. I had been on the clinical service only a few days when I did my first heart transplant, on July 4, 1979. Ed Stinson was the attending on call, and he came in from a Fourth of July party to help me. It was a transformative experience. I took out the swollen, dying heart and dropped it twitching into a bucket. The patient was on bypass. I looked into the empty chest, at a human being without a heart, kept alive by a machine. Nothing I'd ever done matched that moment.

The patient, a physician from Texas, did well. He was the first of twenty-five heart transplants I did over the next twelve months. This was more than half the world's total over that span. To match that today, you'd have to do as many as eight a day, every day. Sir Terence English later told me that after starting his heart transplant program in Cambridge in England, he did eleven heart transplants between August 18, 1979, and July

31, 1980. So, between us, we did three-quarters of the world's transplants during that period. One patient that I transplanted that October in 1979 remains alive and well today and is the longest living heart transplant patient in the world.

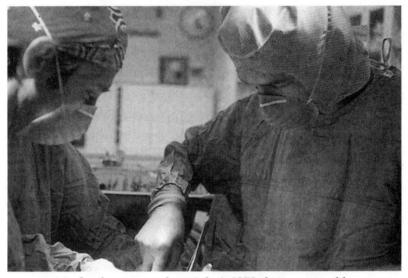

My first heart transplant, July 4, 1979–being assisted by Ed Stinson in his trademark bandana.

Being Shumway's chief resident was hard work but also stimulating and a great privilege. I reveled in it. In addition to transplants, we did two routine heart cases every day in Shumway's room, ten a week—plus emergencies. Shumway would always be present for the main parts of the operation, standing on the patient's left—the assistant's side. He was so good that he could operate from the assistant's side at any time, something that would befuddle many skilled surgeons. He never asked to change places. We would operate together, like partners moving in unison across a dance floor. This was surgery as good as it gets—quick, effective, safe, and fun.

Shumway was great company in the operating room. We would talk about everything—the patients, politics, gossip, the future. He was invariably considerate and generous. Shumway was shorter than me and always asked for a stool to stand on. He could have lowered the table to a height that suited him, which is what all my other chiefs would have done.

I was used to working hard, but now my load was doubled as the transplant chief resident and Shumway's chief resident. While Shumway and I were scrubbing in for a case one day, one of the nurses said, "Dr. Shumway, you've got to let Stuart have some rest."

"One of these days, he's going to get a good long rest," Shumway said with a small smile, "and there'll be nothing he'll be able to do about it." He was making a joke that had an element of truth in it that I understood completely. I wanted to make the most of every minute of what I was doing.

As exhilarating as the work was, I never forgot what was at stake. You might think a heart surgeon works behind a kind of protective wall, insulated from bad outcomes by the knowledge that you're operating on patients with no other option, patients who, if they die in surgery, were already living on borrowed time. If you fail, your failure can be at least partially excused. But I have never felt that way. To me, nothing is more important than making a patient's last hope his or her *best* hope. I became a surgeon to fix people. I always believe that I will—and I am devastated when I can't. It's rare nowadays to lose a patient in surgery. We have so many assist devices to keep someone alive that they usually make it out of surgery. But it can happen, and it used to happen more often. When it did it was awful. You feel drained, almost paralyzed. An inner voice tells you that you just killed someone. Even if the case was hopeless and there was nothing you could have done to change the result, you cannot alter the fact that the patient came into the OR with a beating heart and did not leave the same way. It doesn't matter if the patient would have died the next day. You may have done everything right, but you were still the instrument of someone's death.

I remember everyone I've lost.

....

There was a heart surgeon in private practice who sometimes operated at Stanford who was not part of Shumway's team. He wasn't as good as we were, and Shumway resented him. When a patient came to Stanford for heart surgery, they assumed they were being treated by Shumway's group. Shumway believed this other doctor's poorer outcomes reflected badly on him. When the guy—we'll call him Dr. Smith—disappeared for a time, Shumway turned to a nurse in the middle of an operation.

"I haven't seen Dr. Smith for a while," he said.

"Oh, he's away because his father died," the nurse answered.

"What happened?" Shumway shot back. "Did Dr. Smith operate on him?"

John Wayne, the actor, who lived in Los Angeles, had decided to travel across the country to have a heart valve replacement at Massachusetts General Hospital, ignoring Stanford, which offered the best heart surgery anywhere. After Wayne's upcoming surgery became public, Shumway came into the operating room and was not his usual pleasant self. After a long silence, he said, "I don't care if John Wayne's going to the Mass General to have his heart surgery."

Nobody answered him.

The next day the same thing happened. After staying quiet for a time, Shumway said, "I don't care if John Wayne's going to the Mass General to have his heart surgery." The next day, he did it again. Finally, on the fourth day, Shumway brooded in the OR for what seemed an eternity until he said, "I don't care if John Wayne's going to the Mass General to have his heart surgery, leastways, not nearly as much as John Wayne's going to care!"

Despite the tremendous advances we'd made, heart transplantation remained risky. Outcomes were uncertain. We were still refining immunosuppression regimens and learning how to treat the rare infections we would see in immunosuppressed patients. We weren't yet using cyclosporin in the human patients. All of this meant that we had to be selective about whom we accepted for transplantation, and we had many more prospective patients than we could take.

At first, the upper age limit for a candidate was fifty. Then it rose to fifty-five. Over the years, as Shumway got older, it went to sixty, sixty-five, and then seventy. The patients had to be of exemplary character and have the social and family support necessary to ensure that they would commit to taking their medications for as long as they lived, as failure to do so would be fatal. If a patient had a drug problem or alcoholism, they were out. It was the same for divorced patients, the reasoning being that a spouse was the one person who could ensure compliance with medication. This restriction was lifted over time as almost all the cardiac surgical faculty got divorced. At our transplant meetings, I would look around the room at all the wild, diverse, and immensely talented characters Shumway had brought into the inner circle of his team and wonder how many would pass the stringent tests of respectability we had devised.

A famous film actor from Britain, a household name, was referred to us with end-stage heart disease. He needed a transplant. He had already had unsuccessful coronary artery surgery. We turned him down because he was fifty-four, which at the time was over our limit. He died shortly thereafter. Times change. Today, we have no real age limit. A fifty-four-year-old transplant patient would now be considered relatively young.

I have learned not to look over my shoulder at the past. You cannot live your life backwards. We live now in a medical world no one believed possible a hundred years ago, when you could die of a trivial infection for lack of antibiotics. But I have often thought of that actor. If we had accepted him, he might still have died before we found a donor, or he might have died after his transplant. Nothing was for sure. But he might have lived on, too, perhaps for a long time.

The link between the lab and the clinical service remained strong. We relied on Charlie Bieber's rabbit ATG. Although I no longer had time to do lab experiments, I kept tabs on what was happening. Heart transplantation was considered experimental, and as we were almost the only ones doing it, we were given a lot of latitude to take chances—to try things that would never be permitted now. Our patients had little to lose.

One day Bieber asked me if he could use one of the monkeys to make monkey ATG. He figured that their ATG might work better than rabbit ATG, because they were primates. This made sense, and I told him to go ahead. A couple of weeks later, he came to me with a vial of bloody fluid, his first batch of monkey ATG.

"Let's try it intravenously," he said.

For a second, I wasn't sure what he meant. Then I realized he was talking about giving it to one of the patients.

"Whoa, Charlie," I said. "That stuff looks pretty poisonous. Why is it so bloody? If you want to give it as an IV, let's at least give it to a monkey first."

Bieber went off a little crestfallen. He came back the next day to say it had been a good decision. The monkey he gave it to died overnight. Charlie went back to work and a few weeks later came back to me with a vial of clear fluid. I agreed to give it, but only intramuscularly. It seemed to work. Since there was no adverse reaction, we then tried it intravenously. Again, all was well. We set up a regimen in which we gave the monkey ATG intramuscularly and then intravenously on alternate days. The theory was that the lymph nodes were at least partly responsible for producing the lymphocytes that were rejecting the heart. By giving the monkey ATG intramuscularly, the lymphatic channels would absorb it and take it to the lymph nodes where it could disrupt the lymphocyte factory. By giving it intravenously the next day, we would take out any lymphocytes that were already in the bloodstream. It worked.

We biopsied the hearts of our patients every week. This was my job. A biopsy of the heart muscle gave us early warning of rejection. Every night, after a long day of surgery, I would take one or two of the heart transplant recipients into the operating room, and under local anesthesia, slip the long forceps into the big vein in their necks and down into the heart. I had to be quick, because this wasn't part of my regular surgery schedule. I must have done thousands of these biopsies. I got so I could do one in under ten minutes.

I knew all the transplant patients intimately. In those days, they were in the hospital for two or three months after surgery. Seeing them several times a day, I soon knew everything about them. Late at night, if they were still awake, I would stop by to chat, or to play backgammon with them. One patient I'll never forget was named Betsy. She came to us from San Diego with an inoperable tumor in her heart. The cancer hadn't spread, but because of the tumor's size and location, it couldn't be removed. After some discussion, we decided we should remove the tumor and heart together and do a transplant. Betsy, who was only nineteen, went to work in our office filing and doing odd jobs while she waited for a donor.

Heart transplants are usually done in the night. That's because most donors are declared brain-dead during the day, so it's after dark by the time you've organized a team, harvested the heart, and brought it back. We did Betsy in the night. The tumor had enlarged her heart so much we had difficulty getting it out of her chest. But otherwise the operation came off smoothly. We later wrote up our experience in the *Journal of Thoracic and Cardiovascular Surgery.*

After her surgery, Betsy did well. She was discharged and went home to San Diego. Two years later she got pregnant and called me to discuss the situation. Though she was not married, she wanted to have the baby. No one before had ever had a baby after heart transplantation. I was not worried about the ability of the transplanted heart to support a pregnancy and the delivery. The unknown was whether the drugs she was on to prevent rejection could harm the fetus. Determined to see the pregnancy through, Betsy decided to take the chance. She had the baby, and everything was normal.

Shortly after the delivery, I got a call from a newspaper reporter in San Diego. He asked me if I knew a heart transplant patient named Betsy.

I said of course, she was my patient.

"Do you know she has just had a baby?" the reporter said.

I told him that I did know, and that I'd discussed it with Betsy.

"Are you aware that she is unmarried and she has called her baby Sierra Jamieson?" the reporter continued. "What have you got to say about that?"

I told him to get his mind out of the gutter, and that I was honored that she chose to name her baby after the person who had saved her life. I thought I'd set the record straight, but I should have learned a better lesson about dealing with the press—as I would painfully discover a few years down the road.

Betsy and I stayed in touch. Eventually she developed a tumor in her brain that forced her off her medication. She died of heart rejection. Her daughter, Sierra, was raised by her grandparents. She is now in her thirties and has a family of her own.

Although Shumway was in charge of the entire program and did more general cardiac cases in both adults and children than the other surgeons, I never saw him do a heart transplant or even assist on one during the time I was at Stanford. The transplants were always done by the chief resident, assisted by either Ed Stinson or Phil Oyer in the early days, and later also by Bruce or me.

We had our own cardiac anesthesia group, and our own OR nurses in the cardiac unit. It was a good standard of care that emphasized experience and continuity. When I was chief resident, Bill New was one of the staff anesthesiologists. Bill earned a master's degree in electrical engineering from Stanford, then did his medical training at Duke, followed by a PhD from UCLA. When we were operating together, he spent a lot of time under the drapes that covered the patient, fiddling with a new machine he was inventing. It turned out to be a pulse oximeter.

When he was six, Bill had built a crystal radio set as a Boy Scout project. He loved to tinker. The idea for the pulse oximeter came to him when he remembered how on camping trips as a kid he sometimes put a flashlight behind his hand—which was illuminated sufficiently that he could see the pink color of the blood inside. He turned this into a device that clipped onto the fingertip to monitor oxygen saturation in the bloodstream. When oxygen levels fell, the color changed. After perfecting his invention for a year and a half in our OR, New founded a company to manufacture it called Nellcor. In 1995 he sold Nellcor for $2 billion.

When I knew him, New was just one of the guys helping us get through the difficult problems of the day. Ed Stinson, Bill, and I were sitting around in the surgeons' room waiting for a donor heart to arrive one night. It always took longer than we expected, because livers and kidneys were usually harvested by other transplant teams from the same donor. The teams all came from different places, usually by private jet. Coordinating the donor surgery took time. While Ed and I were talking, Bill arrived with some Chinese food, which he offered to share with us. I eagerly accepted, but Ed just took another draw on his cigarette. "No, thanks," he said, "I get by on Marlboros, a can of Coke, and chocolate cake." It was probably true. I never did see him eat a meal.

Craig Miller joined the faculty when I was chief resident. Miller was a character, a cowboy at heart. He was always in boots and a cowboy hat. Shumway told a story about when Miller was a medical student and first scrubbed in with him to assist on an operation. Shumway noticed a brown stain spreading over Miller's mask. Ignoring this at first, Shumway was alarmed to see that the stain grew until it covered the whole mask. Shumway sent him out of the OR. Miller had never scrubbed before. He hadn't realized that he wouldn't be able to spit out the tobacco he chewed incessantly, and had gone into the OR with a mouthful. After a while he'd felt a little sick and started dribbling the chew into his mask.

In 1980 there were only three cardiac centers in the world doing heart transplants: Shumway's group at Stanford, Dick Lower's group at the University of Virginia, and the bunch at Cape Town. Stanford was the unquestioned leader. We had visitors from around the world who came to find out what we did that they couldn't. The answer was our history—years of dogged laboratory research by which we'd learned to diagnose and treat rejection.

The year flew by. Toward the end of my time as chief resident, Shumway asked what I was going to do the next year.

"Why, sir, I will be going back to the Brompton," I replied.

"Why don't you just stay?" he said. This time he didn't add "for another year."

I told him I would be delighted to. And that was it. I was going to be appointed to a permanent staff position at Stanford. There was no discussion of salary or what my job would be. I didn't know if I'd even have an office. And certainly there was no contract. I just said thank you and we shook hands.

I called Paneth. He didn't seem surprised; I think he had an idea all along that this might happen. He said he was happy for me.

CHAPTER SEVENTEEN
WINNING HEARTS AND MINDS

I joined Shumway's staff at Stanford in July 1980, a year after Bruce Reitz and Craig Miller had come aboard. Counting Ed Stinson and Phil Oyer, I was now the sixth person in the group. Ed and Phil operated in room 12, and Bruce had joined Shumway in room 13. Shumway now generally did the morning cases and Bruce the cases in the afternoon. Bruce was still in charge of the lab, and work continued with cyclosporin and the monkeys. The new chief resident who took over that job from me was John Wallwork, a young English surgeon who had been recommended to Shumway by Terence English in Cambridge. He was coming for a year's fellowship.

Wallwork was a jovial sort and got on well with Shumway, who appreciated his sense of humor. When he arrived, Wallwork was surprised that Shumway never used cardioplegia, a cold solution that is injected into the aorta to stop the heart and preserve it while it was being worked on. Shumway had extensive experience with the use of cold saline applied topically. His method was simply to clamp the aorta and bathe the heart in cold saline that was continuously run into the heart cavity. Shumway's outcomes were impressive, unmatched anywhere in the world. But Wallwork was skeptical. When he first assisted Shumway at an operation, he watched as Shumway clamped the aorta, stopping the heart's blood supply, started the cold irrigation, and got on with the operation. At first, the heart fibrillated, and continued to do so until it got really cold. Sensing that Wallwork was apprehensive, Shumway said, "You see, the heart is getting really cold."

Wallwork, looking down at the quivering, fibrillating heart, said, "Yes sir, I can see it shivering!"

After I joined the faculty, Craig Miller and I shared an office. He was the only one in Shumway's group who had nothing to do with the transplants and had not even looked after postoperative transplant patients as a resident. But he was an excellent technical surgeon. He did every kind of heart operation other than transplants. His main interest, though, was vascular surgery. Shumway made him head of the vascular service and also the cardiac unit at the VA hospital, about ten miles away in Palo Alto. Our office was small, with barely room for two desks. I had to get up and step out to make way for him to get in, and vice versa. Fortunately, we were both so busy that it was rare for us to be in the office at the same time. Craig went on to gain an international reputation as a vascular surgeon, and became the president of the American Association for Thoracic Surgery.

I was assigned to be Miller's number two at the VA and cochief of vascular surgery at Stanford. Of course, I still picked up as many regular cardiac and transplant cases at Stanford as I could. These were usually the night cases. Everyone else preferred to operate in the daytime, and after the sun went down, they were happy to let me take over. I got to be known as the midnight cowboy.

My appetite for heart surgery was never satisfied. I was so hungry for work that one evening when I'd just arrived back in California after an exhausting trip to Europe, where I had been lecturing, I said yes when the chief resident met me at the airport to ask if I could assist on a heart transplant that night. Phil Oyer was on call but said he was sure I'd want the operation. I did. In retrospect, I don't know how I managed to work nonstop all those years. I guess at the time it didn't seem like work.

I made time to keep in touch with the lab, which was close to the office I shared with Miller. We had found that the monkeys with heart transplants did well when we treated them with reduced doses of steroids, coupled with cyclosporin but no ATG. When we tried heart-and-lung transplants, we didn't use steroids at all for the first two weeks, to speed the healing of the airway. The monkeys did fine. The evidence for the effectiveness of cyclosporin continued to mount. Toward the end of the year, we were ready to use it in the patients.

The Food and Drug Administration (FDA) and the Stanford Institutional Review Board gave approval for a preliminary trial of cyclosporin in human heart transplantation. And we had a candidate in mind. In December, a young man in the intensive care unit was dying of a cardiomyopathy, a class of diseases that attack the heart muscle. There was little we could do. He needed a transplant. While we searched desperately for a donor, we tried treating him with a balloon pump, a device that is threaded up the leg artery, in an attempt to augment the heart's output. A few days later, a young girl in another state had an accident that resulted in irreversible head trauma and was declared brain-dead. Although she was smaller than our patient, we decided to take a chance that her heart would work. Phil Oyer was the attending on call, and he asked me to retrieve the donor heart while he started on our patient with John Wallwork. I flew to the donor's hospital and opened the chest. The heart was tiny, almost certainly too small to keep an adult man alive. I called Oyer to discuss the situation. There really wasn't a decision to make—our patient would die unless we did something. We decided to go ahead.

Back at Stanford in the operating room, I scrubbed in to help Phil. When we saw how small the donor heart really was, we knew it wouldn't work on its own. On the spot we decided to sew it in and leave the old heart in place. The donor heart would serve as an auxiliary pump, and the output from the old heart would remain, at least temporarily. Barnard had used this method. His reasoning was that if the donor heart was rejected, there still would be some underlying circulation provided from the native heart. This operation, called a heterotopic transplant, or "piggy-back operation," had not been used before at Stanford. Our focus had been on the prevention and treatment of rejection, not in dealing with its consequences. Leaving the old heart in place, where it would continue to fail and become a source of potential infection or blood clot, did not seem optimal.

But in this case, we really had no choice. As we got the donor heart sutured in alongside the patient's own heart, the new heart took over about half of the cardiac output. In the days and weeks that followed, the donor heart got stronger and progressively provided more of the circulation until the patient's own heart was doing nothing. The man recovered, was discharged from hospital, and lived a normal life for many years with two hearts in his chest. He was the only patient to have a heterotopic heart transplant at Stanford and was the first patient in the world to be treated with cyclosporin for a heart transplant, that December in 1980.

From then on, cyclosporin was the mainstay of antirejection treatment in all the heart transplants at Stanford. We did not change the treatment regimens of the patients who had previously been transplanted and were doing well. In one of the few papers on transplantation that he published, Christiaan

Barnard credited Stanford's development of heart tissue biopsies and the introduction of cyclosporin as the primary reasons that heart transplantation came into widespread use.

In 1981 we were the only program in the world using cyclosporin in heart transplantation. The results were superior. For many drugs, measuring their levels in the body is an essential tool in maintaining the proper dose. But in the early 1980s, there was no assay for blood levels of cyclosporin. We had to learn by trial and error. We started the patients on twenty-five milligrams per kilogram of body weight per day. We knew the drug could be toxic to the kidneys in larger doses. If we saw the kidneys start to fail, we cut back on the dosage. As so often proved to be the case, the trick was to go to the limit of what should be done—and then stop. It seemed to work.

Our improving results with heart transplantation, plus the gains in immunosuppression we'd achieved with cyclosporin, convinced us that it was time to try a heart-and-lung transplant. Only three heart-and-lung transplants had previously been done in humans. Denton Cooley transplanted a two-month-old baby with an otherwise inoperable heart and lung defect in August 1968. The infant lived for fourteen hours. Walt Lillehei, who had moved from Minnesota to New York, performed the second heart-and-lung transplant on a forty-three-year-old patient with bad heart and lung disease in December 1969. The patient did well at first but died of pneumonia eight days later. Had cyclosporin been available to Lillehei, things might have turned out better. A third operation was performed by Christiaan Barnard in Cape Town in July 1971, on a forty-nine-year-old man with severe lung disease. The patient lived for twenty-three days and died from complications when the airway sutures failed. Barnard, unlike Cooley and Lillehei, had chosen to sew the airways separately for each lung instead of connecting the main airway.

At Stanford, we now had long-term survivors among our monkeys that had undergone heart-and-lung transplants. They seemed to be living life normally. These were also the first long-term survivors of lung transplantation. The immunosuppression regimen was working well. We started making a list of potential human recipients. All the patients we initially considered had pulmonary hypertension—high blood pressure within the lungs. As the heart works harder and harder to pump blood to the lungs, it will begin to fail. This is a fairly common and usually irreversible condition that leaves the patient struggling to breathe and the heart damaged. There was no drug therapy for it at the time. Other patients we looked at as possible candidates had congenital heart defects that had not been repaired when they were children because those techniques hadn't yet been developed. Now holes in the heart or sometimes abnormal blood vessels were causing excess blood flow to the lungs and damaging fragile lung arteries. Altogether, these patients had both lung and heart disease for which there was no treatment, but they would certainly die unless something could be done for them.

Bruce Reitz had presented the results of the monkey heart-and-lung transplant work at the sixtieth annual meeting of the American Association for Thoracic Surgery in San Francisco in April 1980. During his talk, he reviewed our laboratory results. Twenty-five monkeys had had heart-and-lung transplants. Five of those monkeys had had an auto-transplant—their heart and lungs were taken out and put back in. One of these auto-transplants was still living seven months after the surgery. Twelve monkeys that had been transplanted with other monkeys' organs but without receiving immunosuppression drugs had lived for at most five days before dying of rejection. Two more had had their own organs taken out and replaced, with the operation done on heart-lung bypass instead of the hypothermia technique. Those animals were still alive. The remainder, also done on bypass, had transplants from other animals and were treated with cyclosporin. The longest survivor (Mom) was still alive nearly four months after the transplant, without rejection, and was doing well. The monkeys who were treated with cyclosporin were the longest-reported survivors after heart-and-lung transplantation at the time.

Unlike Dick Lower's presentation on Stanford's early transplantation research back in 1960, when nobody had showed up to hear him, this new report generated intense interest and some attention from the press. Mary Gohlke, the advertising accounts manager at the *Mesa Tribune* in Arizona, saw a story about our work and wondered whether we could help her. She had been diagnosed with primary pulmonary hypertension and was getting worse. She'd had to stop working when she became so short of breath that she could barely get around. Gohlke had gone to Houston to see Michael DeBakey, a renowned heart surgeon, who had confirmed her cardiologist's diagnosis. He told her she could not be treated. Someone on DeBakey's team mentioned a heart-and-lung transplant but added that such a procedure was still "impossible."

Gohlke was going downhill. She had two teenage sons, and she wasn't ready to die and leave them behind. After reading about our work, she phoned in the summer of 1980 and asked to speak to Reitz. Bruce was polite but noncommittal. He told her about what we had learned with the monkeys, but emphasized that everything was still experimental. He said that heart-and-lung transplantation might be able to help her in the future. He didn't say it, but he must have known her future was going to be a short one.

Gohlke called back several months later. She said her condition had worsened. She wanted to know if we would consider her for a transplant. In October, Mary and her husband, Karl, came to Stanford to meet with Bruce and the heart transplant team.

She was an excellent candidate—and we were her only hope. But we weren't ready. We hadn't yet tested cyclosporin in a human heart transplant. That would have to come first. In early 1981, after several heart transplant patients had received cyclosporin and were doing well, the Institutional Review Board at Stanford gave approval for a combined heart-and-lung transplant in an initial patient. Even though the FDA had approved cyclosporin at Stanford for initial trials in heart transplantation, they had still not approved it for heart-and-lung transplantation. This seemed like a technicality, but without the FDA's approval, we couldn't proceed. Mary continued to get sicker. When she heard that we were waiting on the FDA, she called the editor of her newspaper, who had friends in the Arizona congressional delegation. Arizona senator Dennis DeConcini intervened, and suddenly we had a green light from the FDA. Gohlke moved to Palo Alto to be nearby until a donor could be found. We didn't know how long that would take or how much time we had. When she arrived, Gohlke weighed only seventy-six pounds.

We had not yet done much work on lung preservation for transplantation in the laboratory, because we'd been focused on the operative technique and the subsequent prevention of rejection. We decided to transport any potential donor to Stanford, so that the organs could be removed in room 12 and the transplant done in room 13. This would minimize the time the lungs were out of the body.

Six weeks went by. Mary was fading. Then a nineteen-year-old man was killed in a traffic accident in Southern California. His body was flown to Stanford. Bruce called me that evening with the news that our first heart-and-lung transplant was a go. There was much preparation. John Wallwork was busy getting the consent forms in order, making sure enough blood was available, and calling in the anesthesia and the heart-lung bypass team. Like any team, a surgical crew is only as strong as the weakest link. We were lucky at Stanford that Shumway had gathered an outstanding group of people over the years, and not just the surgeons, but everyone who contributed to an operation, from the anesthetists to the nurses to the intensive-care recovery unit. We were ready now.

The operation began shortly after midnight on March 9, 1981. Ed Stinson and Phil Oyer were in room 12 with the donor. Shumway and Reitz began on Mary Gohlke in room 13. Mary was put on bypass, and her worn-out, failing heart and lungs were carefully removed. We were accustomed to the sight of a totally empty chest in monkeys, but seeing one in a human was different. The heart and lungs were so much bigger. Looking into the empty space where the vital organs should be made us all pause for a second. The heart-lung machine hummed. Mary Gohlke, with no heart and no lungs, was alive.

Stinson and Oyer had removed the donor's heart and lungs so that they would be ready when room 13 sent for them. Shumway was there to take the blame if anything went wrong. This was how he worked, taking responsibility for bad outcomes and giving all the credit to his colleagues when things went well. He set an example I hoped to follow someday. The mood in the OR was relaxed. The surgical procedures had been practiced many times. We were confident it would go well and believed that no amount of additional research could have made us any better prepared.

Phil Oyer brought the donor heart and lungs into the OR where Gohlke was. They'd been flushed and cooled in a bowl of saline exactly as we had done it in the lab. Reitz and Shumway started to sew them in. First the trachea, the main airway, and then the entrance chamber of the heart, carrying the venous blood, and finally the aorta, the lifeline to the body. When all the air had been purged, the flow of blood to the heart was restored. Slowly, it began to beat. Then the lungs were inflated. The heart-lung machine was disconnected. Mary Gohlke was on her own again. Behind our masks, everyone was smiling.

The operation was finished a little before dawn. Security guards were posted at the entrance to the intensive care unit to discourage interlopers from the press. There was a lot of press interest, as this was an operation that had never turned out well before. I don't know what they hoped to report—but I was pretty sure I knew what they expected to report.

Gohlke made slow but steady progress. She was weak from her prolonged illness. She had a lot of ground to make up. Some of the nerves to her stomach had been affected by the operation, and she subsequently needed an additional abdominal operation. Yet she was cheerful. Day by day, she got better. Three months after the surgery, Mary Gohlke—the world's first successful heart-and-lung transplant—was discharged from the hospital. She stayed in the Stanford area for some time to ensure that everything was okay before going home to Arizona, where she went back to work at the *Mesa Tribune.* Gohlke and Max Jennings, the executive editor of the paper, coauthored a book about her experience titled *I'll Take Tomorrow.* Gohlke became an informal ambassador for the Stanford program and took up the cause of organ donation.

We did four more heart-and-lung transplants that year. Two of the patients did not leave the hospital because of postoperative complications. But a new era had begun. The lungs could now be transplanted in a human, bringing hope to thousands of patients with otherwise untreatable lung conditions. Mary Gohlke lived for five more years with her new heart and lungs. She died of complications from a fall. Her heart and lungs showed little signs of rejection.

In the spring of 1982, one year after the Gohlke operation, Bruce Reitz left to become chief of cardiac surgery at Johns Hopkins Hospital. Shumway appointed me the director of

heart and lung transplantation and director of the research lab.
I was thirty-four years old.

....

Now that I was in charge of the laboratory, I wanted to concentrate on what I thought was important to advance the program.
If we were going to expand the numbers of heart-and-lung
transplants we were doing, we would have to find a way to preserve the lungs for an extended period of time when they were
out of the body, just as we could do with the heart. We had
a grant from the National Institutes of Health (NIH), which
we supplemented with money from the clinical program. Dr.
Shumway never restricted our use of these funds, which were
plentiful in those days. Nowadays university hospitals are often
better at counting their money than spending it.

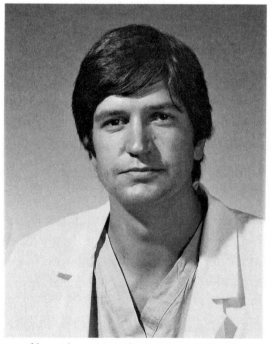

*Director of heart-lung transplantation and the experimental
laboratories at Stanford. I was thirty-four.*

The lungs present a unique challenge. Unlike the other organs, they are exposed to the outside air. Indeed, that is central to their function. They have to transfer oxygen from the air to the blood. The cells that make up that interface are fragile, and their blood supply is unusual. The pulmonary artery, the artery from the heart to the lungs, does not carry oxygenated red blood as arteries do for every other organ. The pulmonary artery carries deoxygenated blue blood—to which the lungs add oxygen. But the lungs themselves also need oxygen, and so in addition to the pulmonary artery they are supplied by the bronchial arteries, which come directly off the aorta and carry oxygenated blood.

I did my first human heart-and-lung transplant in June 1982. This was Stanford's sixth and the world's ninth. The recipient was a young man who had had a previous thoracic operation for a congenital condition. He now had irreversible lung disease and a severely damaged heart. Shumway, who had been present for all the previous heart-and-lung transplants, was out of town. We started the operation in the early evening. Phil Oyer was in the next room with the donor. We were about to learn a terrible lesson.

When I opened the chest, I found that the patient's lungs were embedded in a dense matrix of scar tissue from the previous surgery, which had gone in through the side. It was as if they were cemented in. I wasn't sure I could get them out. New arterial vessels had formed in the scar tissue to supply more blood to the dying lungs. Everything I touched started to bleed. But there was no going back. The patient would die if we stopped. It took forever to get the lungs and heart out, and it was bloody. In the early hours of the morning, I started to sew in the new heart and lungs. That was the easy part. The bleeding from all the raw surfaces continued, and the new lungs were damaged by the repeated blood transfusions we had to give. We worked through the night, but it was hopeless. After twelve hours in the OR, there was nothing more we could do. I was devastated, and so exhausted I could barely stand.

I went home. It was getting light. I collapsed into bed and had barely closed my eyes when the phone rang. The patient's mother, who lived on the East Coast, had flown in and just arrived at the hospital. She had left home when we had informed her that we had a donor for her son. She did not know what had happened after that.

I returned to the hospital to break the news, feeling numb. I explained to his mother that despite our best efforts, her son had died on the operating table. I did my best to comfort her. When I finally went home again, it was hard to put one foot in front of the other. I felt like I was carrying a weight that threatened to crush me.

When Shumway got back, he was entirely supportive. But I could not get over what had happened. I kept going over the experience we'd had with the third patient in our heart-and-lung transplant series, who'd been operated on a year earlier. She had also had previous heart surgery and had also died. Had we missed something? In that case the prior surgery had gone in through the front of the chest and there was no extensive scarring. So it was hard to say whether prior chest surgery was a deal breaker, but I didn't want to take any more chances. I decided not to accept anyone else who'd already had heart surgery. This stayed our policy for many years.

As our transplant list grew, we had to find a way to preserve the lungs out of the body. Bringing a brain-dead patient from far away to Stanford Hospital wasn't practical in the long term. There were rules against transporting bodies across state lines, which forced us to seek time-consuming exemptions from government officials every time we wanted to move a donor over a border. Our goal in the lab was to find a solution with which to perfuse the lungs and make them cold without injuring the delicate exchange cells that make up the fragile boundary between blood and air. A worker's strike at Stanford kept our regular technicians away from work. We carried on without them, enlisting the help of two visiting medical students from Germany. One of these, Hermann Reichenspurner, would in due course go on to be an internationally recognized surgeon in his own right, and the president of the International Society for Heart and Lung Transplantation.

We eventually found a preservation solution that worked on lungs. We also modified our surgical technique to preserve the vagus and phrenic nerves, which control the abdominal organs and the diaphragm, both of which had been damaged in Mary Gohlke's operation. The technique we developed then is still used today.

We still had more people in need of transplants than we had donors. Four months passed as we marked time. Then, in early November, we got word of a donor from out of state. This was going to be a test of our new lung solution. The donor team flew out. When they got to the donor, they flushed the heart as usual and the lungs with the new solution. Everything went perfectly, and lung function after the transplant was normal. The press still followed us closely, and reports of this operation spurred an increase in the numbers of donors we were offered. After a hiatus of four months, we did three heart-and-lung transplants in four days. All the donors were from out of state, and all had their organs removed at the hospitals they were in. All the recipients did well. Lung transplantation had arrived.

I didn't concentrate on transplantation exclusively. In those early years on the faculty, I was busy building up my practice in regular heart surgery, doing valve replacements, aortic surgery, and bypasses. Shumway often asked me to do his cases, too. I kept an eye on his schedule. Whenever I saw he was still in the operating room at five p.m. and I was free, I would scrub in and stand there until he saw me. Then he would leave. Many years later he told me how grateful he was. Nobody else ever did that for him.

We began to see warning signs that lung transplantation might not be forever. A thirty-two-year-old man from Binghamton, New York, named Charlie had been transplanted on May 1, 1981. He was the second heart-and-lung transplant in the Stanford series, and only the second heart-and-lung patient in the world to have been discharged from hospital. He had done well for three years but now suffered from narrowing of the bronchioles, the small air passages in the lungs. This could only be the result of chronic rejection. We increased Charlie's cyclosporin dosage, but this had caused kidney failure. Charlie was soon on a ventilator, which required a tracheostomy, a hole in the neck to access the trachea.

In the heart, chronic rejection is manifested by progressive narrowing of the coronary arteries. We now learned that narrowing of the small airways in the lung was a hallmark of rejection in that organ. Charlie's situation was dire. The only thing that could save him was another heart-and-lung transplant. We doubted this was possible. Charlie's general condition was poor. A re-transplant of both heart and lungs had never been attempted. And our experience with the scarring adhesions encountered in a patient who'd had previous heart surgery told us that Charlie's chances of surviving the surgery were remote.

How much worse would this be in someone who'd had a complete heart-and-lung transplant? Surely both Charlie's heart and lungs would be heavily scarred and stuck to the chest wall. The surrounding nerves that supplied the diaphragm and the abdominal organs were sure to be bound up in this same mess. In the end, we decided we could not use a precious donor for Charlie when we had so many other patients waiting for a new set of heart and lungs. It was a horrible decision to have to make, but we felt it was out of our hands.

Charlie had been on the ventilator for about six weeks, clinging to life, when I got a call from Chris McGregor, Shumway's chief resident. I had begun to wean myself from the unremitting day-and-night hospital schedule I'd kept since my days at St. Mary's, when the best I could do to get away was to stand on the balcony of the entry hall late at night. McGregor's call came on a Sunday, and I was at my ranch in San Gregorio, forty-five minutes from the hospital. He told me we had a donor who was the wrong size and blood type for everyone on the list but one.

"What about doing Charlie?" Chris asked.

If we didn't use the heart and lungs, they would be wasted. Charlie was just waiting to die. I didn't have to think. I told McGregor I was on my way.

We spent the rest of the day doing Charlie's operation. It was the first redo heart-and-lung transplant in the world, and I suspect that even now no more than a handful have been tried. If any. The operation was challenging, but not as difficult as we'd feared. In the earlier case, twenty-five years had allowed the scar tissue and vascularity to build up within the chest. Charlie's chest surgery was much more recent. Everything in his chest was stuck and scarred, but it was manageable. Shumway came in for a while but did not scrub. He just chatted with the nurses and let us know he was around even though it was a Sunday.

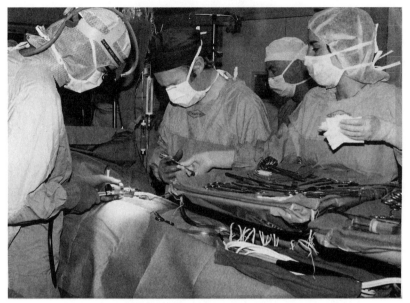

The world's first redo heart-lung operation.
I am being assisted by Chris McGregor (in the dark cap).
Dr. Shumway (in the white cap) is observing.

One problem we had was that the previous donor's trachea was hardened in place, and Charlie's own trachea had been compromised by the tracheostomy that had been done to put him on the ventilator. It was impossible to get back to the original suture line to sew the new donor trachea to Charlie's. So I cut the previous donor trachea and sewed the new one to that. Charlie now had segments of three tracheas—his own, and two from different donors. This worried me. It seemed like a perfect setup for everything coming undone. But there was nothing else for it. I decided that if Charlie's airway didn't fall apart, I would never worry about the sutures of the trachea again. It didn't, and I didn't.

There was another thing I'll never forget about that operation. The day before it, I'd been clearing brush at my ranch and had gotten covered in poison ivy. When McGregor called me on Sunday morning, I was coming out in a rash all over my body. It was driving me crazy. Operating for many, many hours, standing there under the hot operating-room lights as I itched everywhere and could do nothing about it, was torture. As soon as we were done late that afternoon, I tore off my gown and asked the anesthesiologist to give me a shot of steroids. He did, and the relief was almost instantaneous.

Unbeknownst to me, there was a surgeon visiting from Brazil that day who observed the operation. I had friends in Brazil. Soon, I heard from one of them.

"Stuart, is everything all right?" he asked.

I assured him that it was.

"Are you sure?" he persisted. This went on for a while. "You would tell me if anything was wrong, wouldn't you?"

Of course, I said. Finally I asked him what it was all about. He said he'd heard from someone who'd seen me operate that when I finished I desperately needed an injection. He thought I must be a drug addict.

A few days later, when I was in the intensive care unit, Shumway came up to me, put his arm on my shoulder, and said, "That was a terrific job. I don't know anybody else who could have pulled it off."

Charlie recovered, left the hospital, and wrote a book. Chris McGregor later joined the faculty at the Mayo Clinic and became the head of transplantation there.

We were still learning. We continued to monitor rejection of the lungs by doing heart biopsies. We still thought it was likely that since the heart and the lungs came from the same donor, both organs would reject together. But as we'd seen earlier in monkeys, the lungs seemed more prone to rejection. In 1983, we learned that was the case in humans as well. Our thirteenth patient did well for the first two weeks before changes in his lungs showed up on an X-ray. His heart biopsies were negative, so we initially assumed this was infection and not rejection. We gave him antibiotics. After a few days with no response, he was having difficulty breathing. I took the risk of treating for rejection. If I was wrong, any infection would quickly get out of control because of the increased immunosuppression.

It was the right decision, but it was too late. The patient died of rejection of the lungs. The heart showed no signs of rejection. We later were able to show in the laboratory that the lungs could reject independently of the heart. It was another important lesson that had been learned at terrible cost.

Our program kept expanding. For the next year, I headed the only team in the world doing heart-and-lung transplants. We had a big waiting list and were doing an average of one operation a month. Then, in November 1983, cyclosporin was released for general use by the Sandoz company under the trade name Sandimmune. This launched or restarted heart-transplant programs around the world.

In January 1984, I presented a paper on our experience with heart-and-lung transplantation at the opening of the annual Society of Thoracic Surgeons meeting in San Antonio, Texas. The paper was judged to be the most significant of the meeting, and was subsequently published in the *Annals of Thoracic Surgery*. Reviewing our findings for the society, Dick Lower wrote:

> Dr. Jamieson and colleagues report one of the most extraordinary clinical studies of this decade and perhaps of this century. Total heart and lung transplantation combines in one procedure impressive technical expertise with an understanding of complex anatomical, physiological, and immunological principles, a combination perhaps unparalleled in the surgical literature.

That same year, more than fifty centers worldwide started doing heart transplantation, and by 1985 there were more than a hundred. Ten years later there were more than 250. Cyclosporin is still the most widely prescribed immunosuppressant for organ transplants. Shumway's persistence and our determined work in the lab meant that many thousands of people who otherwise would have died of heart or lung disease were given a new chance at a normal and healthy life.

Despite the new enthusiasm for heart transplantation in adults, nothing was happening with transplants in babies and children. Adrian Kantrowitz in New York had done the first transplant in a baby in December 1967, commencing the operation at the same time that Christiaan Barnard was finishing up his landmark transplant in an adult in Cape Town. The infant lived only a few hours. Almost seventeen years later, even with the huge advances in heart transplantation that had taken place, nobody else had transplanted a baby, largely because infant donor hearts were unavailable.

Then, in London on July 30, 1984, Dr. Magdi Yacoub transplanted a heart from a three-day-old Dutch baby into nine-day-old Hollie Roffey. Roffey suffered from a birth defect called hypoplastic left heart syndrome, in which the main pumping chamber of the heart is underdeveloped. Roffey died eighteen days after surgery.

That fall, on a Sunday morning in October 1984, a baby was born in the high California desert who was to make medical history. The five-pound, nine-ounce girl appeared normal, but her heart had the same defect as Hollie Roffey's. The little girl's days were numbered. Her name was Stephanie Fae Beauclair-Drew. Soon the whole world would know her as Baby Fae.

Leonard Bailey at Loma Linda University Medical Center, who headed their cardiac team, specialized in heart surgery in babies. Having seen countless babies die of heart defects that could not be repaired with conventional heart surgery, Bailey had always been interested in heart transplantation in infants. As a medical student, he had visited the Stanford laboratories when that program was just beginning.

Bailey called me in 1983 to ask if I would come to Loma Linda to spend a day with his team. I asked what it was about. He was reluctant to say on the telephone. Curious, I flew to John Wayne airport in Orange County, where Len was waiting for me on the curb. We drove to Loma Linda, about forty-five miles away, through open fields that have long since disappeared beneath California's endless concrete jungle. During the drive, Bailey told me about the work he had been doing in the laboratory during the past several years. At first I wasn't sure I was hearing him correctly. Then I realized why he'd been reluctant to tell me what was going on. At the hospital we walked into a conference room filled with people, including doctors, laboratory workers, and nurses.

The team launched into a presentation of seven years of work on cross-species transplantation in newborn animals. Their research was based on the idea that the immune system is not fully functional at birth. It takes time to develop the antibodies that cause the hyperacute form of rejection known to occur in cross-species transplants—and that I'd studied in the lab back in London. Bailey had performed some two hundred same- and cross-species experimental transplants in the neonatal period, mostly using goat, lamb, or piglet hearts transplanted into baby goats. On average, the transplanted goats without immunosuppression survived about two and a half months before beginning a slow rejection. This was totally different from the rapid, hyperacute rejection I'd observed countless times in mature animals. Bailey's team had a goat named Livingston that had been transplanted with another goat heart as a newborn and grew to six months of age without immunosuppression. It appeared that the immune systems of Bailey's animals were intact, but they were more accommodating as newborns. When the team used cyclosporin, the animals were far less likely to reject the new hearts. Some had grown up and had their own offspring.

We discussed other work that had been done in cross-species transplantation, particularly the work of Dr. Keith Reemtsma, who had transplanted chimpanzee kidneys into human beings at Tulane in the early sixties. He had some success despite the limited immunosuppression then available. But adult heart transplantation using primates had been a dismal experience. Barnard's baboon-transplant patient had died hours after the operation. A second attempt, this time with a chimpanzee heart, failed after three and a half days. Barnard gave up cross-species transplantation because of the rejection issue, though he said that he'd try again when better antirejection drugs were developed. But in a 1978 interview, Barnard said that he'd had second thoughts about ever again transplanting a primate heart, "not because I'm so convinced I'm on the wrong track, but because I got emotionally involved with the chimp."

Among potential animal donors for a human, primates would be best. Chimpanzees were not available, and in any case were so humanlike that nobody wanted to use them. Christiaan Barnard wasn't always wrong. Orangutans and gorillas were endangered. But baboons were plentiful and controlled as pests in many parts of Africa. They are hardy animals and reproduce easily. Bailey's team decided that their donors would have to be baboons.

After they were done talking, I encouraged them to continue their research. I told the team I thought neonatal heart transplantation across close species might be possible. I returned to Stanford intrigued by Bailey's work and the careful way that they had conducted their research. The ethical issues were serious, but I was impressed by Bailey's absolute integrity. And I thought he might well be on the right track.

Sir Peter Medawar, who had won the Nobel Prize in 1960 for his transplant research, and whom I had met when I was working in Ken Porter's lab, had discovered that the immune system is not preprogrammed to distinguish between self and non-self, but learns to do so as a result of exposure during early development. In other words, if there were no preformed antibodies against an organ from another species, there was a chance such an operation could work. Bailey would be taking a huge chance if he transplanted a baboon heart into a human infant, but he was on solid theoretical ground.

When twenty-four-year-old Teresa Beauclair had delivered her baby at a hospital in Barstow, the infant was promptly transferred to Loma Linda for an assessment of a heart defect. The news could not have been worse. Beauclair was told nothing could be done to save the baby. She had three choices: Leave the baby at Loma Linda to die, take her back to the hospital in Barstow to die, or take her home to die. Furious, Beauclair demanded to know why we could put a man on the moon but couldn't make her baby well. She took the infant back to Barstow.

One of the pediatric cardiologists at Loma Linda who'd seen Beauclair found Len Bailey and asked whether he was ready to do a cross-species transplant in a human. When Bailey said yes, the doctor told him he had just discharged a baby home to die. The family lived up in the high desert. He offered to have someone contact them to see if they had any interest. They called Teresa Beauclair, and she agreed to meet with Bailey.

Beauclair brought the baby back to Loma Linda. The father was unable to accompany them, but Teresa recorded the conversation with Bailey to share with him later. According to Beauclair, Bailey discussed his research and emphasized that doing this procedure on her baby, whom he referred to as Baby Fae, would be highly experimental. He told Beauclair he could promise nothing other than without a transplant Baby Fae would soon die. At first, it all sounded like mad science to Beauclair. But she felt she could trust Bailey, and in the end agreed to go ahead. Baby Fae was readmitted to Loma Linda hospital. Dr. Sandra Nehlsen-Cannarella, a respected immunologist at New York City's Montefiore Medical Center, came to Loma Linda to screen the baboons for one compatible with Baby Fae. She found that the child carried no preformed antibodies to baboons, which meant that a hyperacute rejection was unlikely. This was a good sign. Nehlsen-Cannarella supported the operation. Teresa Beauclair, she said, was doing what any mother in similar circumstances would.

Baby Fae was operated on in room 3 of the Loma Linda University hospital on Friday, October 26, 1984. Bailey replaced the small, dark-haired, blue-eyed baby girl's heart with one from a baboon. Baby Fae was twelve days old. At 11:35 a.m. her new heart began to beat spontaneously. Len Bailey called me later in the day to tell me about it. I warned him there was going to be a lot of publicity, but neither of us was prepared for what followed.

The transplant made front-page news in almost every daily newspaper in the United States. The surgery was news in London, Paris, Berlin, Tokyo, Hong Kong, Singapore, Cape Town, and Beijing. Television crews from the major American networks set up satellite trucks at the university. During the first week following the surgery, some 275 representatives of the world press traveled to Loma Linda. Reporters camped out by the hospital and in front of Len Bailey's home.

Reaction to the news was mixed. In an editorial on Saturday, November 3, the *San Diego Union* said, "the great medical team at highly respected Loma Linda University Medical Center has demonstrated medical science at its best, which is to say it was willing to dare failure and controversy to save a life that would otherwise have been lost. And even if Baby Fae does not survive, she and her doctors will have advanced medical knowledge for the ultimate benefit of mankind." That was how I felt. Joanne Jacobs, a columnist in the *San Jose Mercury News*, wrote that she was glad Baby Fae had been given a chance, even against desperate odds. "I wouldn't want to live in a society that let its children die without a fight," Jacobs wrote.

Not everyone was as generous. John Najarian, the chief of surgery at the University of Minnesota—who would have understood an undeveloped neonatal immune system, but who certainly knew little about Bailey's research—said the operation was a mistake. "Everything we know indicates that the heart is going to fail," Najarian said. "The operation will merely prolong the dying process."

I fully expected the crush of press attention, and also the comments of others in the field, both pro and con. But I did not anticipate that picketers would appear at Loma Linda, vehemently protesting the use of an animal to save a human baby's life. The animal-rights people seemed to consider Baby Fae's life no more valuable than a baboon's. Bailey received death threats. Soon the press turned on the parents. They reported that Teresa Beauclair was separated from the father and living a meager existence. They suggested that she lacked the judgment to make a medical decision. Beauclair talked about all of this later. "I may have been young and naive," she said, "but I wasn't dumb. I had feelings."

The ethics of doing an operation that was experimental were also extensively questioned. This struck me as a complete misunderstanding of how medical progress is made. The fact is that *every* medical first is an experiment. Without experimental procedures medicine wouldn't be a science and might still be in the hands of witch doctors and barbers.

Baby Fae did well at first. But she died at nine p.m. on November 15, 1984, at the end of her twentieth postoperative day. Though the exact causes of her death remain incompletely understood, rejection appears to have been a minor contributor. At a press conference the next day, Bailey was tired and drained. Up until then, others had handled the press conferences while Bailey was busy looking after Baby Fae. He had risked his reputation to try to save this child. Now he could only say what he believed. "To cherish the life of one child," he said quietly, "is to value the lives of all. A rescue mission need not succeed to be brave." He went on: "We don't know for sure what happened. I am convinced that we did all we could." Teresa later said, "The night that Stephanie died, I asked Dr. Bailey not to let this experience be wasted, and to keep going forward with it."

That was not to be. I believed that Bailey should carry on. But he was finished with cross-species transplants. The protests and death threats were too much. Hate mail continued to pour in, and Bailey feared for his family's safety. But there was one unexpected happy outcome. The intense coverage of Baby Fae raised awareness of the need for human infant donors. Within a week of Baby Fae's operation, a two-year-old donor became available for eight-month-old Sara Remington, a Houston baby with inoperable end-stage heart failure. Denton Cooley, who had attempted a heart-lung transplantation in a two-month-old in 1968, operated on Remington on November 1, 1984. She lived for another thirteen years.

....

At a 1985 conference in London, I gave a talk on heart and heart-and-lung transplantation. During my lecture, I discussed the experience with Baby Fae. I was on a panel with Denton Cooley afterward. We were taking questions from the audience. Christiaan Barnard stood up, and in his broad South African accent said, "Professor Jamieson, I am surprised that you are supportive of the experiment with Baby Fae, which I consider irresponsible."

I pointed out to Barnard that his first heart transplant could have been considered experimental, and that Baby Fae lived longer than his patient did in that case. The room erupted in applause. Barnard, who was used to being treated like royalty, looked displeased and sat down.

A little more than a year after Baby Fae's operation, a braindead newborn baby who had suffered from asphyxia at birth in Northern California was offered as a donor to Loma Linda. Just three days earlier, a baby boy had been born there, weighing six pounds, with the same condition as Baby Fae—a hypoplastic heart. Bailey transplanted him with the donor heart on November 20, 1985. That child, known as Baby Moses, became the world's first successful newborn heart transplant. I was delighted that Len Bailey could enjoy this achievement. Still, busloads of people opposed to Bailey's latest experiment showed up to picket his house. Baby Moses, whose real name is Eddie Anguiano, is now in his thirties and lives with his family in Las Vegas, Nevada, where he works in one of the hotels. Sometimes an experiment becomes a human life.

Baby Moses was the first of many babies and children whose lives were saved with heart transplants at Loma Linda. Success bred more success, as infant donors continued to increase for the program. Len Bailey had paved the way for a wave of infant heart transplants. By 2011, more than fifteen hundred children under the age of one had been transplanted around the world. Survival rates in children are now the same as those in adults. Bailey, after being publicly pilloried over Baby Fae, is now regarded as a true medical pioneer.

Christiaan Barnard and I were often invited to speak at the same meetings. He talked about heart transplantation, and I talked about cyclosporin and heart-and-lung transplantation. Barnard was a celebrity wherever he went. On several occasions, I heard him end his talk by announcing that he was retiring and that this was the last speech he was ever going to give. This always produced a standing ovation. The last time we were together was at a meeting in Tampa, Florida, in January 1984. He'd retired from active practice the year before but remained a fixture on the lecture circuit. As usual, he ended his talk by saying it was his farewell speech—which was met with the usual adulation. I felt like I'd lived through this one too many times, and afterward I approached him, trying to look both surprised and dismayed. "I'm sorry to hear that this was your last speech, Chris," I said. "But since it was, can I have your slides?"

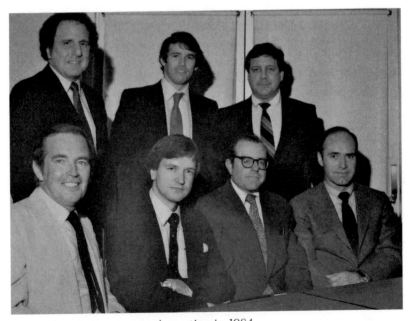

A meeting in 1984.
Bottom row (left to right), Christiaan Barnard, Me, Richard Lower, Bruce Reitz. Back row (middle), Robert Jarvik, designer of the Jarvik artificial heart.

Barnard's jaw dropped.

"Er, well, Stuart, I'll send them to you," he said.

I never received them.

Barnard was replaced as head of the Department of Cardiothoracic Surgery in Cape Town by Bruno Reichart, a surgeon from Munich who rejuvenated the surgical and transplant programs. I'd never liked Barnard, whom I thought was not a good representative for heart transplantation. Reveling in his reputation as a handsome playboy, Barnard had married a series of ever-younger women. He became obsessed with youthfulness and the search for "anti-aging" cures. He signed on as a spokesman for an expensive skin cream that was supposed to get rid of wrinkles. I was always careful about talking to Shumway about Barnard, who had cheated him out of being the first to transplant a heart. But one time, when Shumway was sitting in my office at Stanford, I mentioned what seemed to be Barnard's fear of getting old.

"Did you hear Barnard is promoting an anti-wrinkle skin cream?" I said.

"Yes," Shumway said. "I tried it on my scrotum, and it doesn't work."

I was involved in founding the International Heart Transplantation Society, when these operations were still considered experimental, and before the advent of lung transplantation. In 1980 Dr. Michael Hess, a cardiologist working with Dick Lower in Virginia, suggested we hold a preliminary meeting at the American Heart Association scientific sessions scheduled in Miami in December. Representatives from nearly a dozen cardiac centers showed up, including one contingent all the way from Oslo, Norway. This was encouraging, as only Stanford and two other centers had active programs. This was before the development of cyclosporin and many hospitals and most health insurers considered heart transplantation a waste of resources. The evidence that transplantation was an effective treatment for heart failure was still unpersuasive. Most operations were financed privately or under special arrangements.

Another planning meeting was held the following year in Chicago. I reported that Stanford now had a one-year survival rate for heart transplants of 70 percent. Again, this was before we were using cyclosporin. Nobody else was doing as well, and most cardiac centers were still not doing transplants at all. The board of trustees of the Massachusetts General Hospital had elected not to support cardiac transplantation, and this decision was defended by the *New England Journal of Medicine*. The secretary of Health and Human Services decided not to pay for heart transplants under Medicare. All of which made the idea of a heart transplant society seem off point. But we decided to go ahead, renaming the group the *International Heart Transplantation Society* to broaden the base. We talked about publishing a journal and set up a national registry to track transplants in the US.

Our first formal meeting was in San Francisco in March 1981. About fifty people showed up, including Norman Shumway, Ed Stinson, and Phil Oyer. Shumway was elected the honorary president. The first issue of the journal *Heart Transplantation* came out that summer in 1981. It included a paper in which I reviewed the Stanford experience, including the first eleven patients to have been treated with cyclosporin. I closed on an optimistic note, writing that improved immunosuppressive drugs such as cyclosporin would likely result in greater use of cardiac transplantation. I took over as the fourth president of the society and served a two-year term from 1986 to 1988. By this time the journal was widely read, and the registry had become a valuable resource. *The Journal of Heart Transplanta-*

tion was in due course renamed *The Journal of Heart and Lung Transplantation.*

By the end of the 1980s, the experiment was over. Transplantation of the heart and the lungs had been accepted as valuable procedures and were routinely done to save the lives of dying people with heart and lung disease throughout the world. Cyclosporin and the Stanford experience had made the difference.

CHAPTER EIGHTEEN
ON MY OWN IN A COLD PLACE

The University of Minnesota was a storied institution to me, the cradle of heart surgery. Spanning the banks of the Mississippi River in Minneapolis, the university had been a hotbed of innovation in a frigid location. Under its legendary chief of surgery Owen H. Wangensteen, pioneers like John Lewis and Walt Lillehei had flourished at Minnesota, and they, in turn, had nurtured the generation of surgeons that included Matt Paneth, Christiaan Barnard, and Norman Shumway. The University of Minnesota served as a mecca for those who wanted to develop the field. No aspiring cardiac surgeon could afford not to spend some time in Minnesota. Between 1951 and 1967, Walt Lillehei alone trained more than 150 surgeons from around the world. For me this professional family tree was personal: it was the close relationship between Paneth and Shumway that had brought me to Stanford and to the summit of the transplant world.

But Minnesota's stature in the field of cardiac surgery had fallen. When Wangensteen retired in 1967, after nearly four decades as the chief of surgery, Walt Lillehei applied for the job. Everyone expected him to get it. But Lillehei was regarded by the university administration as a brilliant surgeon with non-existent management skills. The selection committee instead looked beyond Minnesota, hiring a kidney-transplant surgeon from San Francisco named John Najarian.

Wangensteen didn't approve and warned the dean of the medical school that under Najarian Minnesota would enter a dry spell during which its top cardiac surgeons would likely leave, including Lillehei. And that's what happened. Lillehei was swamped with attractive offers from around the country, and not long after Najarian's arrival he accepted a job as chief of surgery and chairman at the New York Hospital-Cornell Medical Center—taking many of the senior cardiac surgeons with him.

Lillehei's departure in late 1967 was acrimonious. Lillehei believed that the equipment in his lab belonged to him, and he informed Najarian he'd be taking it to New York. Najarian said the equipment belonged to the university and that he'd decide what Lillehei could have and what would have to stay. On the Saturday night before he left, Lillehei and a small crew arrived at his lab after dark in three rented trucks. They took everything, leaving behind only a single rose in the middle of the floor.

After that there had then been a succession of cardiac chiefs under Najarian as the program fell apart. By 1980, private heart surgeons in the Twin Cities were doing more heart surgery than the university, the place where it all started.

In early 1984, Shumway talked to me about what had happened in Minnesota. To my surprise he asked if I would consider becoming the next cardiac chief there. Although I was happy at Stanford, I was intrigued. The rich history at Minnesota appealed to me. But I was wary. Stanford was the best heart-surgery center in the world. I ran its laboratory and transplant program. Why go to Minnesota, which had fallen off the map? Shumway thought that the situation at Minnesota could be reversed with new leadership and urged me to at least think about it. I said I would, but the more I did the less interested I was. One thing I loved about California was the warm climate, which was so like what I'd grown up with in Africa. Minnesota was unspeakably cold and dark for many months of the year, a frozen outpost that made London look like a sunny paradise. I finally told Shumway I didn't want to go. He let the matter drop.

Several months later Shumway was scheduled to speak at the Transplantation Society conference in Minneapolis. A few days ahead of the meeting, Shumway told me he couldn't go and asked me to take his place. I didn't think anything of it, as he did this all the time. I always felt awkward giving a lecture to a few hundred people who had come to hear Shumway, but I was used to it. It was August, a pleasant time in Minnesota, and I told Shumway I'd be happy to stand in for him.

"By the way," he said, as though it was an afterthought, "when you're there, why don't you take a look at the job at the university?" I'd been outmaneuvered.

I gave the meeting's opening plenary speech, a notable honor. I still remembered going to a meeting of the society in The Hague as a student, and again to the one in Jerusalem a few years later. I'd been in awe of the surgeons who attended back then. Now they were colleagues. My lecture was well received. Afterward, I visited the university. The campus was lush and lovely in late summer. Students were out lolling on the lawns or throwing Frisbees, and joggers ran along the river roads that flanked the Mississippi, which flowed powerfully at the bottom of a wooded gorge. The Minneapolis skyline punctuated the horizon just beyond the Washington Avenue bridge that connected the campuses on either side of the river, and from which the poet John Berryman had famously leaped to his death in 1972. I had a nice tour and went home thinking perhaps I should reconsider making a move to Minnesota.

A couple of months later, the American College of Surgeons held its annual meeting in San Francisco. Najarian was there, and he came down to Stanford to talk to me about the Minnesota job. I didn't know what to make of him. He was huge, a bear of a man. He had a deep voice and a bad hair transplant. Najarian had played football at the University of California, Berkeley. What I couldn't look away from were his huge, fat hands. I found it hard to believe he was a surgeon. He wore a gaudy gold Rolex watch, the sort of thing nobody in Shumway's group went in for. But he politely asked me to think again about Minnesota, and I promised him I would.

Not long after meeting with Najarian, I got a phone call from Richard Simmons, who I would later learn was Najarian's right-hand man. Simmons headed the search committee for the new head of heart surgery. He asked to come out to see me. Simmons got to Stanford when I was in the middle of a heart-and-lung transplant on a patient who, ironically, had been referred to us by the University of Minnesota. The patient was a redo, and I had to work with scar tissue in the chest. It was a long, challenging operation, and I'd been up all through the previous night with the donor. I met Simmons for dinner. We were interrupted several times with calls from the hospital. It was difficult to concentrate on Simmons's sales pitch. Simmons seemed impressed by my concern for a patient. I found it strange that he thought this was remarkable.

I asked Simmons what it would take to rebuild the program at Minnesota. He said that expanding private cardiac practices outside the university were the main problem. I knew this to be true. After Lillehei's departure, the university had taken another big hit when Demetre Nicoloff left. Nicoloff had done his residency at the University of Minnesota Hospital under Wangensteen and then trained under Lillehei. He went on to develop the St. Jude heart valve with Manny Villafana, a brilliant pioneer in medical technology. Nicoloff, then an associate professor, implanted the world's first St. Jude heart valve at the university in 1977. The St. Jude valve went on to become the most commonly used artificial heart valve in the world. A year later Nicoloff performed Minnesota's first heart transplant. But Najarian refused to promote Nicoloff to full professor and also diverted income from the cardiac center to other areas of the surgery department. Nicoloff left the university in 1979 and founded Cardiac Surgery Associates, which practiced out of several competing hospitals. Nicoloff's group soon eclipsed the university's ailing cardiac program.

It's not unusual for good surgeons to become disgruntled with university practice and its attendant politics. Nicoloff's history with the university seemed predictable and unimportant. As Simmons explained how Nicoloff had become the university's main competition, I didn't pay close attention. I should have.

I agreed to make another visit to Minnesota. Simmons sent me an itinerary for three days of meetings. I drove to the San Francisco airport on a Sunday evening after spending a glorious sunny California day at my ranch in San Gregorio. I made my way to the departure gate for a Northwest Airlines flight to Minneapolis. The waiting area was full of people with pale faces who were carrying heavy coats. I sat there looking at them. And then I got up, went back to my car, and drove to Stanford, where I called Simmons.

"Oh, you missed the plane," he said.

"No, worse than that," I replied, "I'm not coming."

Simmons was not pleased. I told Shumway the next day that I had decided not to go. Shumway said that was fine, and that he was happy if I was. "Onward and upward," he said.

....

Shumway once told me that you can tell how good a job is based on who takes it. Over the next year, a number of other candidates looked at the Minnesota job. None took it. It seemed that the challenge was too great, that cardiac surgery at Minnesota was beyond saving. At Stanford, I had been promoted to associate professor and granted tenure. My future was secure. And I loved my work, which now included regular visits from bright young researchers from overseas who came to spend a year or two in the laboratory. We were publishing good papers on the pioneering research we were doing in transplantation and lung preservation. By any measure that mattered to me, I had it all.

And yet I felt dissatisfied somehow. Shumway was only sixty-two in 1985, and unlikely to look for a successor any time soon. There was no longer any way for me to advance. I had plateaued. I was haunted by the words of Matsuo Basho, a seventeenth-century Japanese poet who advised, "Do not seek to follow in the footsteps of the men of old; seek what they sought." I began to realize that staying at Stanford would not be enough for me.

At a meeting in South America that year, I discussed the Minnesota position with Aldo Castaneda, who had left the faculty at Minnesota in 1972 to become chief of cardiac surgery at Boston Children's Hospital. Castaneda had done some early work in heart-and-lung transplantation in baboons while he was at Minnesota. He had been the first to demonstrate that primates did not have the post-transplantation breathing problems that showed up in dogs. We had a long talk over lunch. Castaneda thought the situation in Minnesota could be turned around but stressed that it was *fundamental* that I have complete financial independence for the cardiac unit. He said "fundamental" more than once.

At the end of 1985, a little more than a year after I had backed out of the visit to Minnesota, I called Simmons. I asked him if I could take another look. He was suspicious, but he told me to come. And this time I went.

I had already decided to accept the position. But I had conditions. It was essential for me to have an independent cardiac practice, one that was not controlled by Najarian and the Department of Surgery. I wanted the money we made to stay in the cardiac unit. I had to be able to recruit some new surgeons. Finally, I needed to continue my research and have space in which to do it. What I really wanted was a separate building housing the clinical cardiologists, the surgeons, and the pulmonologists, which I would call the Minnesota Heart and Lung Institute. Simmons seemed to think this was ambitious on my part, but he agreed to all my demands. So did the dean and the chair of medicine—and John Najarian.

When I got home, I wrote to Najarian agreeing to go to Minnesota on the understanding that I would found and lead a new entity, the Minnesota Heart and Lung Institute. I specified that my cardiac surgery group needed to be financially independent of the Department of Surgery. I asked that no promotions of existing faculty be put through before I took up the post. He wrote back agreeing to all of it. I got ready to leave Stanford.

Before my departure, the dean of the medical school at Stanford sent for me. I hardly knew him. I had never been to his office and wondered why he wanted to see me. On entering the room, my trepidation increased when I saw the vice president of the university sitting there. They invited me to sit down. The dean asked if there was anything he could offer to make me stay at Stanford. I told him I didn't think so.

"What about Shumway's job?" he said.

I was taken aback.

"What does Dr. Shumway think about that?" I asked.

"We haven't talked to him about it yet," he responded.

"This conversation's going no further until he's in the room," I said and walked out.

I found Shumway in his office. I told him what had just happened. It was inconceivable to do otherwise. He was furious and stormed off to confront the dean.

I never had another conversation with the Stanford administration.

Saying goodbye to Stanford, and especially to Shumway, was hard. He had been like a father to me. He said again how happy he was for me and how he looked forward to what I would accomplish at Minnesota. He showed me the letter that Matt Paneth had written to him in 1977 asking if he would take me on.

"I don't know if you can afford to take him," Paneth wrote, "but I will tell you this: You cannot afford not to take him."

I drove out of Palo Alto. I was the new chief of cardiac surgery at the University of Minnesota and a full professor. I was going to open the new Minnesota Heart and Lung Institute. I was thirty-eight.

....

I thought three days on the road in my loaded-down Honda Civic would give me time to get used to the idea of being in Minnesota. The Civic was something of a joke at Stanford. Everybody in Shumway's group drove some kind of high-end sports car, except for Ed Stinson, who drove a truck. Craig Miller had once asked me to park at the far end of the lot outside the cardiac surgery offices so as to not let the side down.

I spent the night in a motel in Needles, a small town in the Mojave Desert and the last stop in California before crossing the Colorado River into Arizona. I left California with a pang the next morning and drove on through Arizona, New Mexico, Texas, Oklahoma, Kansas, and Iowa. It was a surprise to find that the highway in many places was lined with billboards advertising for Jesus. I covered more than two thousand miles in two days. I did stop in Tombstone to visit Boot Hill, its famous cowboy cemetery. I liked the idea of men who fought and died with their boots on—not flat on their backs in a hospital, something with which I was all too familiar. I figured I'd be in for a fight in Minnesota and believed I was ready for it. I had no idea.

I bought a small town house a block from the hospital, to be close to my patients. I moved in, and the next day, in early March 1986, I was at the hospital. Some of the patients waiting on the Stanford list for heart-and-lung transplants who lived closer to Minneapolis than Palo Alto had come with me to Minnesota, with Shumway's blessing. There was work to do.

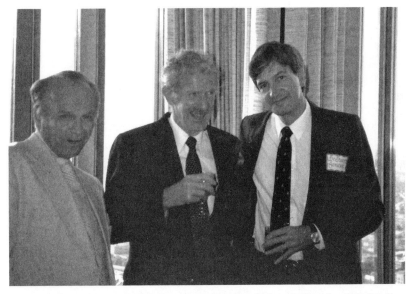

My arrival in Minnesota, 1986. With Walt Lillehei (left), who did the first open-heart operations using cross circulation in 1954, and F. John Lewis (center), who did the first open-heart surgery in the world on Jaqueline Johnson in 1952.

One patient who came with me to Minnesota was a twenty-eight-year-old woman named Barbara. She had been a marathon runner, but now had pulmonary hypertension—high blood pressure in the lungs. It's like putting your thumb on the pulmonary artery. It forces the heart to work harder and harder to pump blood to the lungs, and it becomes enlarged and then progressively fails. Then the kidneys and liver begin to fail. The patient wastes away. The cause of this type of pulmonary hypertension isn't known. Today we can treat it with drugs, but back then a heart-and-lung transplant was the only hope. Barbara arrived in Minnesota with her husband. They were looking for a place to live and I had a guest room on the lower level of my town house, so I invited them to move in with me. It wasn't a good decision. Every night when I came home—if I did come home—they'd be waiting expectantly, wanting to know if a donor had been found. They'd already waited several months, and she was fading.

One night I happened to be at home. Barbara's husband ran up the stairs crying and told me she had collapsed. I went down and found her in bed, on her side. I turned her over, and it was obvious that her heart had stopped. That's what happens in the end with this disease. The heart simply cannot continue to work against the pressure in the lungs and it arrests. And once it does, there's nothing to be done. You can't restart the heart because the problem that caused it to stop is still there. But I commenced CPR anyway, mostly to make the husband feel that something was being done, though I knew it was hopeless. I told him to call 911, and in a few minutes the paramedics arrived and after assessing the situation sent for someone to take the body away. The husband moved out a few days later. I think he was angry with me. I never took in a patient again.

From the beginning, things were different to what I was used to. Most of the good heart surgeons were gone, having either left the state or joined Nicoloff's group. There was practically no heart surgery being done at the university—something I already knew. When I checked on my promised lab space, I learned it still belonged to a member of Najarian's group—who refused to get out. Nothing happened in his lab, but the guy wouldn't move. I didn't want to make waves so soon, but I wanted what I had been promised. When I spoke to the dean about it, he told me to talk to Najarian. Najarian said there was nothing he could do. I strongly suspected that Najarian could do anything he wanted to. But I decided to let it go and leave my research for later while I worked on building up the clinical practice.

Going into the OR at Minnesota was like going back in time. Surgery was being done the same way it had been twenty years earlier. It was like exploring a canyon in the desert and coming upon dinosaurs. Times had changed, but not here. One thing that especially troubled me was that the scrub nurses were not assigned exclusively to the cardiac unit. One day they'd be assisting on a heart surgery, the next they were in the OR for a brain operation. This was not the accepted standard of care. In heart surgery you need the same people there all the time, so they learn the procedures, which are complicated and have to be executed precisely. Every day I'd explain what we were going to do, and in what order, and with what instruments, and what was expected of everyone involved. The next day I'd have to go through it all again. It was like building an elaborate sand castle at the water's edge on the beach. When you come back the next day, it's gone.

It was the same with the anesthesiologists, which was even worse. The chairman of anesthesia had been there since the times when Lillehei and Lewis were in the OR, when cardiac surgery had grown out of general surgery. He didn't see the need to change. Time had passed him by. I began to get a sense of what kind of struggle I faced. I had always worked in hospitals that were on the cutting edge and were striving for excellence. Minnesota was fossilized.

My main hope was that a new university hospital that was scheduled to open in a few weeks would change the environment. Or at least allow me to change it. The new hospital included two cardiac operating rooms. I soon discovered the new setup was less than ideal. It takes a lot of bulky equipment—including a heart-lung machine—to do open-heart surgery. In most hospitals, the biggest ORs are usually reserved for cardiac surgery. Najarian had designed the operating suite in the new hospital. The biggest operating room had been reserved for him. I looked over the rooms I was being given and decided I could make do.

The Phillips-Wangensteen center was the largest building in the university hospital complex. Thirteen stories high, with two additional floors below, the building housed the Department of Surgery and Najarian's lavish office. Jay Phillips was a philanthropist friend of Wangensteen. The son of Russian Jewish immigrants, he had started a liquor business in Wisconsin that became the Phillips Distilling Company. Phillips moved the company to Minneapolis in 1935, and by the end of World War II, the company was the largest spirits distributor in the United States. Phillips's close friend and administrator of his empire was a man named Stanley. I had been in Minneapolis only a few weeks when Stanley was admitted to another hospital in town with chest pain.

In his eighties, Stan had severe coronary artery disease. I was asked to operate on him. I didn't want to operate in a hospital where I'd never worked and didn't know anybody. I persuaded Stan to be moved to the university over the weekend and scheduled surgery for Monday. Stan would be to be our first cardiac case in the new hospital.

On Saturday night, Stan developed sudden chest pain and then suffered a cardiac arrest. Fortunately, I was in the hospital at the time. He was resuscitated, and I put in a balloon pump through his leg to augment his cardiac output. I decided to do the surgery right away. I called in the operating room staff, and we started in the early hours of Sunday morning. By three a.m. we had Stan on the heart-lung machine with his heart stopped. Suddenly, the power went out. Emergency lights came on in the OR right away, but the heart-lung machine did not restart. Unless we could do something, Stan would be brain-dead in minutes.

My chief resident started to crank the heart-lung machine pump by hand. This wouldn't work for long. A technician went off to search for the fuse box and found it in a passageway. A circuit breaker had tripped. When he reset it, the power returned, and I finished the operation with no further interruption.

Stan recovered and became a friend and supporter. It was a start.

....

I had not been in Minnesota long when I got a surprise. Demetre Nicoloff called, inviting me to lunch. How odd, I thought. The devil himself! I met him at the University Club, a quiet, elegant place on storied Summit Avenue, a street where F. Scott Fitzgerald once lived and which curved along the bluff high above St. Paul. We had a pleasant talk. Contrary to what I had been told, Nicoloff did not have horns or a forked tail. He was extraordinarily decent. At one point he asked me what I thought of Najarian. I told him I felt that we got along well, and that I trusted him.

"I hope you never find out anything different," he said and changed the subject. I should have seen this as a warning.

Nicoloff offered to help me any way he could and wished me luck in rejuvenating the cardiac program at the university. I was delighted to have a new friend.

After only six weeks in Minnesota, I did my first heart-and-lung transplant. It was on a Thursday, the first of May. At that time heart-and-lung transplants in the United States had only been done at four cardiac centers: Stanford, where most of them had been done by me; the Texas Heart Institute, by Denton Cooley; Johns Hopkins, by Bruce Reitz; and in Pittsburgh, by Bartley Griffith. This was going to be the first heart-and-lung transplant in the Midwest. The surgery created a stir. There were television crews outside the hospital that I was fortunately able to avoid. I had not yet trained anyone to do the donor operation, but by chance my friend Bruno Reichart, from Cape Town, was visiting at the time. Bruno agreed to supervise the donor team.

The patient was Kenneth Jones, a thirty-seven-year-old Minnesotan—about the same age as me and the father of a six-year-old son. Jones had originally been referred to me at Stanford by the Mayo Clinic. He'd been on the list for six months and had come home to Minnesota when I moved there. Ken suffered from pulmonary hypertension. The donor was a young man who had shot himself.

During the operation the telephone in the operating room rang repeatedly—an interruption I always hated. I told a nurse to turn the phone off. Somehow it kept ringing anyway. Finally, the nurse picked it up. She said a man on the other end insisted on talking to me. I walked over to the phone and the nurse held it up to my ear. The person on the line identified himself as the hospital's chairman of the human subjects committee. He said that the operation I was doing was experimental and that I did not have permission to proceed. I told him that I didn't consider it experimental, but that in any case we had already started and the patient's useless heart and lungs had been taken out and were lying in a bucket. He told me to put them back. I nodded at the nurse to hang up the phone. I went back to work wondering if I'd made a powerful enemy. This absurd demand should have been a warning.

As the operation continued, Najarian came in to watch. I told him about the phone call. He laughed it off and told me not to worry. We started at ten a.m. and were done by three that afternoon. I stayed at the hospital that night to be close by. As I was doing rounds in the intensive care unit, I happened to see Najarian on the evening news. He was talking about Ken Jones's heart-and-lung transplant, although he played no part in it. I was amused, since he didn't do heart or lung surgery, let alone do heart and lung transplants.

Jones did well postoperatively but then developed difficulties with bronchospasms. We learned that the donor had a history of asthma, which we had failed to discover during the workup. The asthma in the transplanted lungs went away after a couple of weeks. Since the nerves between the new lungs and the brain were no longer connected, the asthma that occurred after the transplant indicated that local nerves or muscles within the lungs contributed to the condition. The disappearance of the symptoms signaled that the brain was more important in most patients with asthma. Ken was discharged after three weeks. He is still alive and we have grown into our sixties together. Ken is now the world's longest living lung-transplant patient, and his son now has a family of his own.

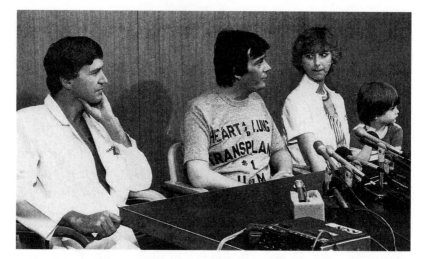

The Midwest's first heart-lung transplant at a press conference six weeks after his May 1986 surgery. I am on the left with Ken Jones, his wife Debbie, and their son. Ken is still alive and well—the longest living lung transplant patient in the world.

Our second heart-and-lung transplant was in a thirty-three-year-old woman from North Dakota named Dee Sellden. Sellden worked in the audit department of the Internal Revenue Service. She had Eisenmenger's syndrome, irreparable blood-vessel damage in the lungs that resulted from a heart defect that could not be operated on when she was younger. Sellden had been a so-called blue baby. Her congenital heart condition mixed her venous (blue) blood with her oxygenated (red) blood. This caused her skin to turn blue. Replacing both her heart and lungs could fix the problem. Sellden's donor was a twenty-one-year-old woman from Fargo named Janis Thompson. Thompson was a premed student and cheerleader at North Dakota State University. She had died after striking her head when she fell while practicing a human pyramid.

After she recovered from the surgery, Sellden was pink for the first time in her life. She marveled at the ruddy color of her fingernail beds and lips, which had always been a dusky hue.

Ken and Dee were the start of our new transplant program, which took off. Our fifth heart-and-lung transplant was in an eight-year-old girl named Cindy. Only Denton Cooley had attempted the procedure in such a young patient, and that was years before and it hadn't worked. But Cindy came through the operation fine, as did all of our other heart-and-lung patients. She left the hospital after three weeks, with her collection of stuffed toys, the youngest surviving heart-and-lung transplant recipient in the world.

As glamorous as the heart-and-lung transplant program was, we did many more heart transplants. We did seventy of them in 1986 and 101 in 1987, making us the busiest heart-transplant program in the world. We achieved another milestone on August 7, 1987, when we became only the third center in the country to be certified to do heart transplants in Medicare patients, which had finally been approved. The other two were Shumway's program at Stanford and Richard Lower's in Virginia.

My main focus, however, was general cardiac surgery, which I believed was the key to building up the center. I started bringing people in. Carl White and Bob Wilson came from the University of Iowa, joining the cardiology team as chief of clinical cardiology and chief of the cardiac catheterization laboratory, respectively. They were joined by an enthusiastic new member of the cardiology faculty, Bruce Wilson. Michael Kaye came up from the Mayo Clinic in Rochester to direct our research efforts and help with donor runs. Paneth sent over a surgeon named Bob Bonser for a year. And I promoted a talented young surgeon who'd been training with me, Jolene Kriett, to the surgical staff. Kriett was one of the most naturally gifted surgeons I'd ever seen—everything she did was instinctive and perfect. She was truly that rare person who was born with a knife in her hand. You can tell by the way a surgeon throws a stitch, and whether the next one comes in one fluid motion, whether they're a natural or not. Jolene was a natural. Matt Paneth used to joke that he could teach a chimpanzee to do heart surgery—and he had done so on several occasions. Jolene had skills you cannot teach.

But at the outset, before I had that kind of help, I did most of the complex cardiac surgery myself. Doing three or four cases a day, I was in the operating room before it got light out and usually left it late at night. I also did operations at other hospitals, sometimes stringing them together one after the other, so that as I finished one patient another one was being opened up on the other side of town. Then it was a mad drive across town. This was before cell phones. The logistics were often daunting.

Two or three times a week, after a long day in the OR, I climbed into the university's small propeller plane and flew to outlying hospitals and clinics in Minnesota, Iowa, North Dakota, or Wisconsin to meet with doctors and tell them about what we were doing at the university. Sometimes I'd give a talk over dinner, often to only a handful of people. But the referrals to our program grew exponentially, and I kept at it. The hardest thing was the weather, which in the winter was brutal. I had never experienced such cold. I learned for the first time that 40 degrees below zero is the same in Centigrade and Fahrenheit. Also that temperatures like that are painful. I had to wear a scarf over my face so it didn't hurt when I breathed.

I came back from these trips late at night to face a mountain of paperwork and a long list of phone calls to be returned the next day. I usually slept in my office. The one break I allowed myself was to get back to my ranch in California for a long weekend once a month. It was like being in another country. So many things in Minnesota were foreign to me. I had to learn to keep my car inside the garage at night in the wintertime, otherwise it wouldn't start in the morning. On one of my first winter mornings, I heard a disconcerting thump-thump coming from the wheels as I drove the first few blocks. It turned out that the tires had frozen and were flattened where they had rested on the pavement. The noise went away once they warmed up.

Returning to Minneapolis on Sunday nights after a trip to the ranch, I felt I almost needed a passport. It was exhausting, but by the end of my first year, the number of open-heart cases done at the university had more than doubled.

On April 10, 1987, just over a year after my arrival, we had the formal opening of the Minnesota Heart and Lung Institute. I invited many distinguished guests. Lillehei was there with his two assistants from the historic first cross-circulation operation. Earl Bakken, the founder of the pacemaker company Medtronic, attended, as did Stan, Phillips's friend. Together they announced an endowment to provide fellowships for visiting surgeons. Norman Shumway and Matt Paneth were there. Matt, who came over with his wife, Shirley, had not been back to Minneapolis since the mid-fifties, when he had been a resident with Shumway under Lillehei. I had chosen a motto for our institute—"Anything Is Possible"—and had a plaque made to hang in the lobby, where I passed by it every day. I believed those words, never pausing to consider that "anything" didn't necessarily mean something good.

We had not yet done a lung transplant without the heart, and few had been done in the world. Joel Cooper in Toronto had pioneered single-lung transplantation and had done a handful successfully. There was almost no experience yet with double-lung transplantation. But I was sure we could do it. We started a waiting list of potential recipients, putting forty-four-year-old Keith Papachek at the head of the line. Papachek had emphysema. His chest was barrel shaped because his lungs were overinflated after years of struggling to breathe.

On New Year's Eve 1987, I was doing my fourth case of the day, taking a clot out of a heart, when Bob Bonser put his head through the operating room door at 6:40 p.m. and said that it looked like we had a double-lung donor for Keith. The donor, from Indianapolis, had suffered a brain injury and then gone into cardiac arrest. They worked on his heart for an hour with CPR and managed to resuscitate him, but his heart was unsuitable for donation. I told Bonser we could talk when I finished.

As soon as we came off bypass, I found Bob. He told me that we now had another donor, this time a heart donor in Chicago. We had a patient who needed a heart. He'd come in with heart failure after a massive heart attack. To save his life, we had put in a temporary left ventricular assist device, a pump that took over much of the work of the heart. This was early days for that technology, and the patient was one of the first it had been tried in. I was not comfortable leaving him on the machine for any length of time. Now, unexpectedly, we had a heart for him. Things were about to get busy.

The logistics were complicated. Mike Kaye, who usually went on the donor runs, was in the hospital with a detached retina. To complicate matters, teams from other hospitals were in Chicago to harvest the kidneys and liver from that donor and had already started. If we were going to use the heart, we had to leave immediately. We also had to harvest the lungs for Papachek in Indianapolis by four a.m., because the donor's funeral was scheduled later that day. I left Jolene Kriett to finish the case I had been working on and headed for the airport with Riyad Tarazi, a cardiac surgical fellow who'd come to us from the Cleveland Clinic. As soon as Jo finished the current case, she and Bob Bonser were to start getting the heart patient with the assist device ready for his transplant operation.

Tarazi and I got to the airport at nine thirty p.m., less than three hours after Bonser had stuck his head in the OR to let me know something was up. The Citation jet had its engines running. We climbed in, closed the doors, and were airborne in minutes, headed for Chicago. Life Flights have air clearance that supersedes all other flights except for Air Force One, the president's plane. On arrival in Chicago, we were met by an ambulance and rushed to the donor hospital with siren blaring and lights flashing. The operation there was uneventful. We cooled the heart, took it out, placed it in a cooler with ice, and were soon at the airport. The New Year had commenced.

We were back in Minneapolis and in the OR by two thirty a.m. I changed into fresh scrubs, relieved Jolene, who'd already taken out the assist device and removed the failing heart. Jolene and Luis Fragomeni, an old friend who'd come to Minnesota as a visiting professor, left for Indianapolis. They were airborne by three a.m. They had planned to grab an hour and a half of sleep on the way, but the heating system on the plane went out shortly after takeoff. Both surgeons were dressed in scrubs with light cotton jackets, and it was bitterly cold. They were still shivering when they reached the donor hospital. As in Chicago, there were other teams there to harvest different organs, and they'd begun. The lungs were exposed, moving rhythmically up and down on the ventilator. Fragomeni checked the blood gases, looked at the condition of the lungs, and told the donor coordinator, "Call Minneapolis and tell them it's a go." The call came through to room 14, my operating room, as I was doing the heart transplant.

We had finished the heart transplant by six a.m. At seven, Keith Papachek was wheeled into the operating room and put to sleep. Jolene and Luis were back in the air, accompanied by a cooler that contained a pair of lungs. The clock was ticking, because the lungs were getting no blood. Starting my seventh operation in the past twenty-four hours, I picked up a scalpel and opened Papachek's chest.

Right away I knew we were in trouble. Papachek's lungs were stuck to the inside of his chest. It would take a slow and deliberate dissection to avoid subsequent bleeding problems. We put him on bypass so that we could collapse the lungs to make it easier to take them out. I had removed only one when Jolene and Luis arrived in the operating room at nine a.m. The donor lungs had been out of the body for three and a half hours, the outer limit to which we had gone before. I had to make a decision. Should I put them in immediately, which meant taking the other lung out quickly and risking bleeding? Or should I take my time when, in fact, we were already out of time? I thought about all those hours in the lab at Stanford we'd spent working out how to preserve and transport lungs. I decided to go slowly.

When I at last got the other lung out, I immediately started sewing in the new ones. Five and a half hours after they had left the donor's body, they were in Keith Papachek's chest. We started ventilating the lungs and shut off the heart-lung machine. Everything looked good. Soon Keith had pink, oxygenated blood running through his arteries, and he was functioning on his new set of lungs. His oxygen levels were normal. We had just completed one of the world's first double-lung transplants, and in doing it had shattered the record for how long lungs could be preserved outside the body. It had been my longest New Year's Eve.

Three weeks later, Keith Papachek went home. Remarkably, his chest had returned to its normal size. In medical school we'd been taught that the barrel-chest signature of emphysema was a permanent change in bone structure. But that turned out to be wrong. Once normally functioning lungs were in place, the chest shrank back.

We had accomplished a lot in the nearly two years I had been in Minneapolis. We had started a heart-and-lung transplant program and built up the busiest heart transplant program in the world. But numbers weren't the best part of the story. By 1988, our one-year survival rate for heart transplants was 97 percent. The new year was off to a great start.

CHAPTER NINETEEN
EXILE

Our clinical practice soared. But I began to understand why so many others had left the University of Minnesota's cardiac program. The problem wasn't fierce outside competition at all. It was something that emanated from within. The more I operated, the more I was resented. The general surgery staff whined that I was taking too much operating room time. An even worse transgression was that because I operated seven days a week, I usually missed Najarian's Saturday morning "grand rounds." Everyone was expected attend to these sessions and to listen to Najarian holding court. My absence was noted, and word got to me that Najarian was offended. He took it as a personal affront that I was more interested in my patients than in hearing him talk.

All of the key promises made to me when I agreed to take the job had been broken. Before I arrived Najarian had appointed someone who had wanted my job to a full professorship—something I had specifically said would be unacceptable. Naturally, this person fought every new idea and technique I proposed. I never got my research space. I hadn't even been reimbursed for my moving expenses, and being too busy to complain, I was perceived as weak for letting it go.

But the biggest disappointment was that Najarian did not give me the financial independence he had guaranteed—the one thing that Castaneda had warned me was "fundamental." Without controlling our own money, we couldn't reinvest in the program. Instead the money went elsewhere. Whenever I went to see Najarian about it, he told me that we would have financial independence as soon as I "knew the ropes." Every month we turned checks over to Jim Coggins, Najarian's financial controller. Every month they got bigger. Soon, we had transferred millions of dollars to Najarian and his group, the Department of Surgery Associates. Ostensibly part of the university, DSA functioned more like a private practice. Coggins was the bagman.

I kept asking Najarian where the money was. He insisted it was in a safe place, and I could tap into it whenever I wanted. He said he knew "to the penny" the amounts he had in all of his department's accounts. But he never gave me an accounting. Our money disappeared into a black hole. When I hired new faculty, Najarian told me how much I could pay them. I thought the pay was low. When the staff complained, Najarian shrugged and said that I set the salaries.

Then there was the Lillehei matter.

Walt Lillehei had returned from Cornell to St. Paul, Minnesota, in 1975, where he became the director of medical affairs at St. Jude Medical. He'd been through a tumultuous time after being convicted of tax evasion and was no longer licensed to practice medicine in Minnesota. In the eleven years since he'd come back, Lillehei had had no connection to the university. I thought that despite his troubles, this was wrong. Everything I'd done in my career was traceable back to Lillehei. I considered him a legend and believed he still had much to offer. I went to see Najarian to ask if I could make Lillehei an emeritus professor.

Najarian's office was an imposing place, a glassy aerie high up in the Phillips-Wangensteen Building. The views overlooking the Mississippi were spectacular, and the walls were lined with photographs of Najarian with the many celebrities he'd cajoled into posing with him. Although there was a comfortable sitting area, Najarian always remained imperiously behind his desk when he met with me. It was the kind of throne room that Shumway would have never dreamed of having. As we talked about Lillehei, I could tell this subject was still an open wound. Najarian told me the story about the raid on Lillehei's lab and the solitary rose. As he talked, huge tears rolled down his cheeks.

Gradually, he composed himself. I argued that Lillehei would help restore prestige to the university, thinking to myself that maybe he'd see this as a credit to himself. I said that there was already money being raised to endow a chair named for Lillehei, a position I would be honored to hold. When I mentioned money, Najarian seemed to lighten up a bit. He told me to go ahead.

I returned along the maze of tunnels to my offices and called Lillehei right away. He was thrilled. I had arranged for his office to be in the institute, and he soon settled in. He was a great asset. Apart from the support and help he gave me, he was an extraordinary teacher and often accompanied us on rounds. He introduced me to Jacqueline Johnson, the first open-heart surgery patient in the world. We were now both thirty-nine.

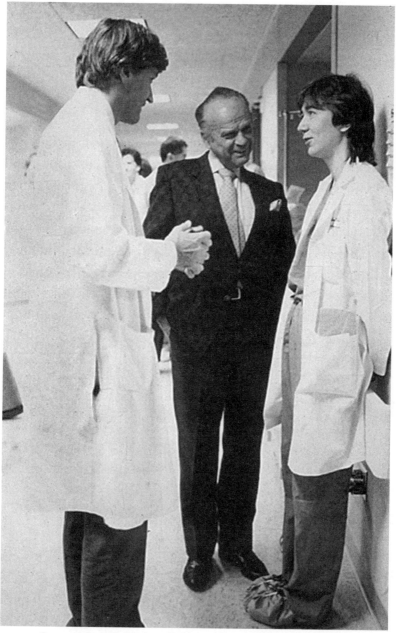

On rounds with Walt Lillehei, and the gifted Jolene Kriett.

A few weeks later, Najarian sent for me.

"I remember agreeing to give Dr. Lillehei an emeritus position," he said. "However, I don't recall allowing you to give him an office." I was dumbfounded at Najarian's pettiness. I told Walt I needed the space and I was sorry, but he would have to move out. I figured it would be better if he thought it was my idea and not Najarian's.

Najarian gave no indication that we would control our own money any time soon, even though two years had gone by and I certainly "knew the ropes" by now. We kept turning over checks to DSA. We had our own accountants, and I talked to them about what to do. I said I didn't think Najarian had any intention of ever giving us control of our money. In that case, they said, why don't you simply stop giving it to him? I hadn't thought of that. But it was an easy call. We opened an account and started making deposits.

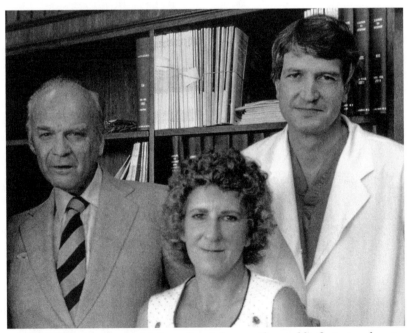

Walt Lillehei and me with Jaqueline Johnson, the world's first open-heart surgery patient when she was five years old. She and I were now thirty-nine.

About a month after we'd stopped handing over checks to Najarian, I was summoned to his office. David Brown (the dean of the medical school) and the CEO of the hospital were there. I had no idea what it was about. The meeting lasted an hour. Najarian had a list of crimes I'd supposedly committed. One claim was that I hadn't hired a nurse because she was too fat, which wasn't true. Another was that I'd stolen the key to the operating room. I didn't even know the operating room could be locked—though if it could have been, possibly one of my staff borrowed a key to get in and would have assumed that there was more than one key. Another charge was that I had misappropriated departmental funds. This was partly true. I had wanted a small gun case for my town house and asked Jim Coggins where I could buy one. He said he knew someone who could get me one. And he did. It wasn't anything special and only cost a few hundred dollars. Coggins paid for it with department money and neglected to tell me that—or to send me a bill. I was busy in the OR night and day and simply forgot about it. I think now it was a setup, something for Coggins to have in his back pocket for future use.

This went on. It was all so trivial and absurd that I couldn't believe the three most important people at the hospital were sitting there talking to me about any of it. At one point Najarian claimed to be exhausted, said he couldn't go on, and handed the list to Brown to continue.

I am sure that I made mistakes, that I was arrogant and demanding at times. I chafed at rules that didn't make sense. One example that came up involved heart valves. You'd be surprised how many patients ask if they can have their old valve after it's been replaced. The rule was that any tissue removed from a patient had to go to pathology, but I'd ignore that and give the patient the valve. Why send it to pathology? So the pathologist can say, "yes, that's a heart valve"—and charge a fee for it?

It would take me longer to figure out what my real crime was. I'd failed to grasp that you could not be seen as better than Najarian. Mediocrity was the key to survival at Minnesota. Najarian was on top, and I was about to find out how far he'd go to stay there.

My mother's sixtieth birthday was coming up. I was scheduled to fly to England, where she and Philip now lived, the day after the meeting in Najarian's office. Everyone knew I was going. Maybe that explains what happened the next morning.

It was August 2, 1988. I woke up to find my picture on the front page of the Minneapolis *Star Tribune*, beneath a headline saying that I was the subject of an investigation. According to the article, I was accused of ordering a coronary-bypass operation on a patient who was clinically dead—plus a second procedure shortly afterward on the same patient, supposedly to control bleeding. The article stated that the surgeon had terminated a procedure that was underway when the patient died, but that I then insisted the surgery be continued. The story went on to suggest that all of this had been done to collect $22,000 from the patient's insurance company. The article quoted a pathologist who said that the surgery was unnecessary, though it did not say how a pathologist would know anything about it.

That wasn't all.

The story also reported that I had covered up an incident in which a pair of forceps had been left in a patient's chest after surgery. The claim was that I told nurses in the OR that a second operation was required to control bleeding, when in fact it was so the forceps could be removed without informing anyone, including the patient's family. The article said it wasn't clear whether I had left the forceps in or someone else had done it. Somehow, X-rays of the forceps inside the patient's chest had gone missing. The bill to the insurance company in that case was $19,000.

I stared at the paper in disbelief. None of it was true. I remembered getting a call from a reporter recently asking me to comment on whether an operation done by my group might have been unnecessary. I'd declined to say anything and forgot about it. Now the timing couldn't have been worse. I'd be in England by the end of the day.

When I got to the office, my secretary was already there, going over the newspaper article. Jolene Kriett—one of the most composed people I'd ever known—was sitting at my desk sobbing.

"What are we going to do?" she asked.

"Jo, we're going to do what we always do," I said. "Work hard." Angry and in shock, I was sure it would not take long for the truth would come out. The story in the paper was so sloppy I couldn't understand how it had been published. I hadn't started to wonder yet where the story had come from. The phone rang all day with calls from reporters. I didn't take any of them. But Jo did.

On August 3, the *St. Paul Pioneer Press*, the *Star Tribune's* competitor across the river, reported that Kriett told them the report was false. The story said that Kriett "angrily denied" that a useless surgery had been performed on a dead patient. She said she was certain because she had done the surgery herself. She told the paper that not only had I not ordered her to do it, I didn't even know about the operation and hadn't been in the hospital when it took place.

Jolene told me hours after the surgery what really happened. The operation had not been bypass surgery. The patient was the mother of young children who'd been brought to the hospital in critical condition after a heart attack. She'd had a cardiac arrest, but was resuscitated with CPR. Considering the young age of the patient, and after consulting the family, Jolene and Carl White, the chief of cardiology, had decided to place her on an assist device. Even though they didn't know if her brain was still functional, they wanted to give her the benefit of the doubt. When she did not regain consciousness, they discontinued life support.

The *Pioneer Press* article reported that Jolene and other doctors said the implication that an unwarranted surgery had been performed for financial considerations was outrageous. And several staff members who'd been in the OR for the other alleged incident said that they saw no forceps during follow-up surgery to relieve internal bleeding. The reporter had also spoken to a doctor—unidentified but one more knowledgeable than the *Star Tribune's* sources—who said it would have been impossible to conceal the discovery of a pair of forceps in a follow-up surgery. The unnamed doctor went on to suggest that the story had been planted to discredit me, probably by "someone with a grudge against Jamieson, a newcomer who has helped quadruple the hospital's cardiac and lung surgery caseload in the two years since he arrived from Stanford University."

Any heart surgeon could have told the *Star Tribune* that it would be impossible to leave a pair of forceps—which are the length of the heart itself—inside someone's chest and sew them in. The story would have been funny if it weren't so awful.

The hospital was in an uproar. I met with the dean, David Brown, plus Najarian and the hospital's director. I told them I was worried the false accusations would destroy the hard work of the past two years. I said I was sure it would all get straightened out shortly. And then I made a big mistake. I offered to stand aside as chief until an investigation was carried out. I did not appreciate that the fix was in. I asked that the investigation be done by outside experts. In the moment it seemed to me the only honorable course of action. But as I would soon learn, I was not dealing with honorable people.

On August 4, two days after its initial story, the *Star Tribune* published a front-page retraction, signed by its executive editor, Joel Kramer. The brief mea culpa said that the paper should not have reported the story.

"Publishing the account of the events, when we had not confirmed it with anyone who had firsthand knowledge of the facts, was a serious lapse in journalistic judgment, which we regret," Kramer wrote. Also on the front page that morning was a story reporting that I was temporarily stepping down as the university's cardiac chief. The juxtaposition could not have been more striking. And when the *Star Tribune's* ombudsman, Lou Gelfand, weighed in on August 7, he wrote only about how the paper had made an "error," gliding past the fact that it was a mistake that could well destroy my career. Gelfand wrote that the reporter had pursued the story after getting a "tip," but he did not speculate on whether such a tip might have come from someone with an ulterior motive. On the contrary, my situation didn't seem to bother Gelfand in the slightest. The only hand-wringing at the *Star Tribune* was over how its mistake had made them look. One sentence in Gelfand's piece said it all. "How," Gelfand wrote, "did the paper get in this mess?"

How indeed? Who was behind the tip? Who had a grudge against me? In a blur of follow-up stories that appeared in the wake of the retraction, the *Minnesota Daily*, the campus newspaper, talked to Arthur Caplan, the director of the university's Center for Biomedical Ethics. Pushing aside the false accusations, Caplan said this was a classic case of cutthroat academic medicine. "It's not unusual for an internationally prominent surgeon to be at the center of a controversy," Caplan told the paper, "because they play in a high-stakes world and our expectations are enormous. They are powerful, and that breeds envy, rivalry, jealousy and turf fights, so difficult controversies swirl around these men."

I had to wonder what he knew.

When I got back from England, I gave Najarian a list of six surgeons for the investigation. The list included Denton Cooley from Texas, and the chiefs of heart surgery at Yale and the Mayo Clinic. All were internationally known and respected leaders in the field. Najarian selected none of them. Instead, he chose two friends who chaired surgery departments, as he did, plus a third person I had never heard of.

I had been in touch with Shumway throughout the ordeal. When I told him the names of the people who would do the review, he said, "We're in trouble." I still didn't want to believe him. But I was soon set straight. A surgeon named Ed Humphrey had been installed in my place while I was suspended. Ed was chief of surgery at the local Veterans Administration hospital. He'd been around for a long time and seemed to know what was going on with my situation. He came to see me, and after we'd talked a little he got to the point. Humphrey said that he'd been told that if I would give up financial control of the cardiac center, and turn over all the money to Najarian, then "all my problems would go away."

It wasn't hard to connect the dots. I told Humphrey I wouldn't do it.

I still had operating privileges and patients who were counting on me. Shortly after talking with Humphrey, while I was in the OR one day, Coggins had the locks changed on my office. A patient waiting inside to see me wondered what was going on and had to be let out later. My parking permit was also revoked. Then, a few days before my review, I ran into a cardiac surgeon I knew in the corridor. I didn't have to ask him what he was doing there. Before the investigation even started, Najarian was interviewing prospective replacements.

The review was set for early September. The night before it took place, Najarian took the committee members out to dinner. They all belonged to the same professional societies he was in. They were cardiac surgeons but not active ones. I didn't know any of them.

I was the first to be interviewed the next morning. They gave me a half an hour. I answered all their questions and asked that I be allowed to meet with them again at the end of the day to respond to any issues that came up in subsequent interviews. I had submitted a list of people from my group I thought should be questioned, but only some of them were. Najarian decided who would be called in front of the committee, and his list was a closely guarded secret. I waited all day to be called back. I never was. Najarian later told me that the committee had had no additional questions for me.

In hindsight, I know the outcome was never in doubt. The facts that I thought would exonerate me were simply ignored. Najarian sent for me a week later and said the review committee had recommended that I not be reinstated. I knew that's what he wanted. I couldn't believe any other reasonable person would agree.

I'd underestimated Najarian's determination to not be eclipsed on his own turf, to rule his kingdom and collect his tribute. I'd been naive. At Stanford, Shumway had protected me—protected us all, like an umbrella, shielding us from university intrigue, never letting territorial feuds or arguments about money come near us. I'm sure there were politics there, but I'd never seen them.

Now I was out. I still had my academic appointment, but I knew I was done in Minnesota. I was forty.

When I finally saw the report of the review committee, it made for interesting reading. It said the creation of the Heart and Lung Institute—the thing I'd come to Minnesota to do—

had been "disruptive." The only thing it had disrupted was the long period of malaise when few cardiac patients were referred to the university. I was criticized for not doing research. This could not have been further from the truth. When Najarian reneged on his promise of lab space, we'd rented space off-campus. In two and a half years, my group had published 148 papers, more than all the rest of the surgical staff combined. After declining to interview most of the people who worked for me, the committee also criticized my leadership style.

There was one charge I could not deny: the committee faulted me for not attending Najarian's grand rounds.

Two weeks after the review, eager to move on, Najarian announced that my successor as chief "may be named within a month," though it was no mystery as to whom it would be. It was the man I bumped into in the hallway before the reviewers came.

....

It was a bitter time for me. I'd been in the right, but the damage to my career and my reputation was real just the same. The future looked bleak. I had enemies now who would work to undermine me wherever I went. What was most difficult for me to accept was that my reliance on honesty and loyalty, instilled since early childhood in Rhodesia, and reinforced by men like Matt Paneth and Norm Shumway, had not carried the day. But one thought kept my spirits up. The people who'd brought me down had no honor. Like hyenas, they were mean and dangerous, but not worthy of contempt.

I heard from colleagues, all of whom offered support. Shumway was unwavering. I got letters and phone calls from Bruno Reichart, Denton Cooley, Sir Terence English, and Len Bailey. They'd all run the press gauntlet before. A friend named Charlie Moore in San Antonio, Texas, may have put it best.

"You're the proof of that old Texas saying," Charlie said. "The higher up the tree you climb, the more people there are shooting at your behind!"

I filed a lawsuit against Najarian's group, the Department of Surgery Associates, and another one against the university. I also sued to find out who had fed the newspaper the story. The *Star Tribune* argued that I was a public figure, and therefore fair game. But they eventually settled out of court. So did Najarian and the university.

In time, things caught up with Najarian, Jim Coggins, and the dean of the medical school. Within a few years Najarian and Coggins lost their jobs and the dean resigned his position. Najarian's department was exposed as a cesspool of criminal misconduct after raids by the FBI and IRS. Najarian was indicted by a federal grand jury on seventeen counts of fraud, theft, and tax evasion. Charges of conspiracy and obstruction of justice were added. Two members of Najarian's staff pleaded guilty and gave evidence against him. Coggins died before he could be indicted and was named an unindicted coconspirator. He had been operated upon by Najarian's new cardiac team and died shortly after surgery. Walt Lillehei, who had never gotten along with Coggins, called to tell me about it. "They're so short of patients now that they've started operating on each other," he said. "Pretty soon there won't be anybody left."

Though it is still published, the Minneapolis *Star Tribune* filed for bankruptcy and entered a long period of decline, shedding many reporters in the process.

But all of that was a long time ago, when I lived in a place where some hearts were irredeemably cold. I moved on.

CHAPTER TWENTY
CALIFORNIA
CALLS

I had immediate inquiries from other hospitals and private practices in Minneapolis. But I wasn't interested in competing with the program I'd built at the university. It would have seemed too much like revenge, which I believe is a self-destructive instinct.

I knew that wherever I went, I wanted to stay in academic medicine. That may seem strange, given that I'd been victimized by academic politics at their worst. But all of my work had begun with research and continued with experimental procedures. These could only be done at a university hospital. And I had another reason. I'd put together a great team at Minnesota and I wanted to take them with me. I was looking for a package deal.

In October, the month after the review, Dr. Moossa, the chief of surgery at the University of California, San Diego, called. He knew about what had happened at Minnesota and asked whether

I wanted to discuss the possibility of coming to San Diego. I said I would meet with him. Although he had a general idea about the situation in Minnesota, Moossa didn't know what was true and what wasn't. He wanted to be cautious. He suggested we meet on neutral ground at the airport in Chicago.

We talked over lunch. Moossa asked about Minnesota, and I asked about San Diego. Heart surgery is the driving force in a surgery program, because of the money it generates, and because of the high visibility of a successful cardiac unit. Moossa was eager to build the cardiac program in San Diego. I liked him. He seemed like a straight shooter. He told me everyone called him Babs. Moossa was born in Mauritius and spoke with a French accent. He had trained in England, just as I had, but he understood that political infighting that was more common in academic surgery in the United States. He said that what we did was a "a contact sport." Moossa had spoken to one of the reviewers who'd investigated me in Minneapolis, and who had recommended that I not be reinstated there. Apparently, this same person told Moossa that he should hire me.

Moossa said his main problem at UCSD was outside competition. I'd heard that one before, but I listened and tried to keep an open mind. Moossa's chief of cardiac surgery was a man named Pat Daily. I'd heard of him. He'd been at Stanford about ten years before my time. Having trained with Shumway, he was a good surgeon. Daily left Stanford for San Diego in 1973, when there was no significant competition there, and established himself as the top heart surgeon in town. But Daily had divided loyalties. He had a thriving private practice outside the university, at Sharp Memorial Hospital. This was in direct competition with his practice at the university. The clinical chief of cardiology at UCSD, who was Daily's age and a friend of his, also saw patients at Sharp. Many patients with insurance, after being first seen at the university, ended up having their surgery at the private hospital. That left the university cardiac unit mainly with children, and adults who had no money or insurance. This was not sustainable. Worst of all, when Daily started a program in heart transplantation in San Diego in 1986, he did it at Sharp Hospital, not at the university, which would have been the obvious choice. Moossa had no doubt which institution Daily preferred. He earned a great deal of money at Sharp while keeping his smaller but steady salary at the university. Moossa told me he wanted to bring all this to an end. That meant finding a chief of heart surgery who would be dedicated to UCSD and who could grow its practice and expand it to include heart-and-lung transplantation.

This sounded good. San Diego might be the right place to start over—and to bring along important members of my team. As it stood, I felt that I'd left them in an untenable position.

Moossa proceeded methodically, still careful to keep a lid on our negotiations. After our initial meeting in Chicago, he asked me to fly to the Los Angeles airport, where I had lunch with him and Michael Stringer, the CEO of the UCSD hospital. Later, I met again with Moossa and the chief of medicine at UCSD, Steve Wasserman, in San Francisco. Moossa then asked if he and Mike Stringer could come to Minneapolis. He wanted to interview my staff at the university himself, with Stringer present. I said that he could meet with whomever he wanted and asked him to send me a list of the people he wanted to see, which he did. Moossa wanted to interview the operating room nurses, the other nurses who worked directly for me, all of my surgical staff, plus all the cardiologists and pulmonologists. These were the people I'd urged the review committee to talk to if they really wanted to know what was going on in the cardiac unit. I arranged everything and reserved a suite for Moossa at a Minneapolis hotel for the interviews. I met Moossa and Stringer at the airport in January. Stringer, who had never been out of Southern California before, arrived in shirtsleeves. It was minus 30 degrees outside. I had to lend him my overcoat.

The meetings went on for two days. Moossa and Stringer must have interviewed forty people. In the end, they went home satisfied that I was their man. The next step was for me to meet with Gerry Burrow, the dean at UCSD, and Richard Atkinson, the chancellor. I had some conditions before we went any further: I wanted to bring my transplant coordinators, Ann Hayden and Becky Robert; the chief of my laboratory, Michael Kaye, who also edited the *Journal of Heart and Lung Transplantation* and maintained the International Registry of Heart and Lung Transplants; plus two surgeons—Jolene Kriett and Riyad Tarazi.

I stayed in La Jolla, at the historic La Valencia Hotel. At breakfast one morning, the waiter, who was from Mexico, looked perplexed. I asked him if anything was wrong. He said he didn't know what to make of the strange white substance on his windshield when he gotten into his car that morning. I realized he had never seen frost before. I took it as a sign that this was the place for me.

Moossa and I talked about salaries, office space, and laboratory support. A nonnegotiable condition was that I be allowed to build a cardiovascular center at the university. All of this was agreed to—though the money was a problem at first. The dean told Moossa that the salaries I had requested were impossible. I would be being paid more than anyone at the university ever had been. I told them that if they wanted the best surgeons in the world, they would have to pay the going rate. Finally, the dean acquiesced.

There was no written agreement, no contract. I remembered how worthless Najarian's letter promising me everything in Minnesota had turned out to be. We shook hands, and that was it. I have never had cause to regret my decision in the nearly three decades since I made it.

It was not all plain sailing. Najarian—who despite his tender ego was powerfully connected—phoned Moossa and promised to make things difficult for him if he hired me. Najarian hadn't merely wanted me gone—he wanted to bury me. Moossa ignored the threat. Then three senior professors in San Diego threatened to resign if I was appointed. They were Daily's friend the chief of clinical cardiology; the head of pulmonary medicine, a powerful, nationally known person named Kenneth Moser—the same Ken Moser who years before had worked with Charles Hufnagel; and Dick Peters, a well-known thoracic surgeon and senior professor who would be on my team if he stayed. They went to see the dean.

When Moossa learned of the revolt, he stood his ground. "Let them quit," he said. Peters had a contact in Minnesota, Richard Varco, a retired professor who still meddled in university politics. Varco had supplied Peters with stories about what a terrible person I was. Shumway had told me that Varco had always been jealous of Lillehei.

My appointment was announced. Nobody quit after all. Then, two months after I started, I found a letter from Dick Peters on my desk. He had sent copies to Moossa and the dean. I went over to Peters's office and asked what it was all about. He told me that Moossa had said that if any of Varco's stories turned out to be true, I would not be hired. Moossa offered to pay Peters's expenses to go to Minnesota and find out for himself—which he did. The catch was that if Peters came back convinced that I was okay, he would write me a letter of apology. So he did. And he became an ardent supporter.

....

But none of this happened right away. Before I moved to San Diego, I went back to Africa to clear my head. I was still shaken by what had happened in Minnesota, mistrustful and wary. I was sure Africa would set me right. I had three months.

I contacted Bruno Reichart, who had taken over as the cardiac chief at Groote Schuur Hospital in Cape Town after Christiaan Barnard retired. Under Bruno the cardiac center was thriving. He also worked at the Red Cross children's hospital in Cape Town, where all the open-heart surgery in children was done. I asked him if he could use a hand, and he said yes, of course. I left for South Africa.

We worked mainly at the children's hospital, a remarkable and rewarding experience. There was a waiting list of several hundred children who needed heart surgery. Bruno and I operated there two or three days a week, whittling down the waiting list. It felt wonderful to be back in the OR. When we weren't working on children, we did transplants and regular heart surgery at Groote Schuur Hospital, where Bruno had caused a stir by insisting that blacks and whites be cared for in the same wards.

The memorial to Cecil Rhodes was nearby, on the lower slopes of Devil's Peak, the hill above Rhodes University. Rhodes's wooden bench was still there, facing northeast where Rhodes had imagined his Cape-to-Cairo railway would start. Sir Herbert Baker designed the memorial, a horseshoe of pillars at the top of a huge staircase. There are forty-nine stairs, one for each year of Rhodes's life, flanked by eight bronze lions. I visited it often.

And every evening, after a long day in the OR, Bruno and I would climb Table Mountain to watch the sunset together, deciding the route when we got there according to our moods. It was three thousand feet to the top, where the air was fresh and you could look out one way over the Atlantic Ocean and the other direction over the Indian.

The anesthesia at the children's hospital was generally administered by a stern, middle-aged German woman. One day, in the middle of an operation on a small baby, I peered over the sterile operating room drapes and noticed that she had blood all over her hands. "I'm surprised that you don't wear gloves," I said.

"Now why on earth should I wear gloves?" she asked.

"Aren't you afraid of AIDS?"

She replied that there were only three cases of AIDS in South Africa, and all had come from "American-tainted blood" through transfusions. I couldn't believe a highly trained doctor would be so misinformed. By 2007, just eighteen years later, an estimate of six million people—or 12 percent of the population in South Africa—had HIV/AIDS. When children were excluded, the rate was over 18 percent, and the total number of people infected was larger than in any other country in the world. The numbers are even higher now. The other top five countries with the highest HIV/AIDS incidence were all neighbors of South Africa. In Botswana, the total numbers are fewer, but nearly half the population is estimated to be infected.

After working with Reichart for two months, I decided to go home—to my real home. I caught the plane that took me to Zimbabwe, back to Bulawayo, and got off at Gate 5, the only gate there was.

....

When I got to Whitestone, after having a look at Raigmore, I drove around to the chapel where Philip and my mother were married and where I had been a choirboy. Someone was practicing the piano inside but stopped when I came in. It was the headmaster's wife, Sally Harris. She told me that the school had been deserted and closed during the civil war. After the war it was renovated and reopened. Now there were five hundred pupils, more than four times as many as when I was there.

The next morning I renewed my acquaintance with the Matopos Hills, driving out along the old road, which looked as

I remembered it. As I drove past places where my childhood friends used to live, some of their houses now fallen down, I wondered what had happened to them. I had lost touch with them all.

The Matopos Hotel that used to stand on a hilltop over-looking the dam had vanished. Even the road leading to it was gone, probably a casualty of the war. The Matopos was a dangerous place to be during the insurgency, just as it was during the Matabele rebellion almost one hundred years before. The sailing club from which I used to sail on the Matopos reservoir was still there, but behind a barbed-wire fence.

I went to Rhodes's grave and World's View. It was as it had been. There is a native taboo against the desecration of resting places. Though his statue had been torn from the cities and many streets were renamed—not to mention the country itself—nothing at World's View had been touched. Leander Starr Jameson was there, too, still lying peacefully, next to the Allan Wilson memorial containing the bones of those who had died alongside him. I sat in the shade of the memorial looking out over the expansive Matopos game park and reflected on the years and events that had passed by since I last was in this quiet place. Rhodes died at forty-nine. I was forty then and wondered what the next nine years held in store for me.

I visited some of the old caves I used to explore. It was a sad business. Since independence, the government had decided to varnish over the bushman paintings to preserve them. But the varnish had turned opaque, casting the paintings in deep shadow. In places, attempts to remove the varnish had removed the paintings as well. What had lasted for thousands of years had been erased in a flash of ignorance and carelessness.

I drove to the Maleme dam and reservoir, which were also unchanged. Signs reading "Beware Bilharzia and Crocodiles" had been posted. Bilharzia is a waterborne parasitic disease.

We all had it as kids. Crocodiles sunned themselves along the shore, just as they had when we used to fish there. I drove out through the game park. I saw giraffes in the distance, and some antelope. Then I came upon a rhino, which was close. I stopped the car to stay with him awhile. He was grazing, oblivious to my presence. During the afternoon, I saw half a dozen more rhinos, including a mother with a calf standing in the rushes next to a stream. The calf frolicked about like a puppy. I watched them from a lookout platform that had been built by the friends of a man called Smith, who was killed at twenty-six in the Rhodesian Civil War. The dedication plaque read, "On active service."

Everywhere I went, I found that no one, white or black, was bitter about the war, which was talked about openly. I was delighted that the game parks were as strong as they ever were, though this wasn't the result of any conservationist impulse. Tourism had become an important industry, and tourists came to see animals. Anyone without a Zimbabwe passport was charged a higher rate when they checked into a hotel.

Back in Bulawayo, I walked the streets, thinking the town was much smaller than it had been when I was growing up. I drove out to the cemetery to visit my father's grave. It was hard to find. There were many more graves now. I finally discovered my father's behind a hedge that hadn't been there before. I stood by it for a long time. I wondered how my life might have gone if he'd been around to give me advice. I smiled when I recalled that he had insisted on being buried instead of cremated, saying that he might need his body in the future. Maybe the fact that I felt compelled to visit him there was what he had in mind.

I took a plane to Victoria Falls. I had wanted to go by train, in a plush carriage behind a steam engine, but I was told that the train was no longer reliable. Though it was sure to arrive eventually, nobody could say on which day. I did see an advertisement for locomotive drivers that said, "No experience necessary."

The pilots on the plane were white, the flight attendants black. Though no black people were onboard, the flight attendants explained the safety procedures first in Shona and then in Ndebele. A much shorter version followed in English. The in-flight beverage service featured warm Coke. As we approached the Victoria Falls airport, I saw a burned-out plane, a Dakota, on the runway. Just as we were landing, we took off again and circled once before coming in at last. No explanation was offered, and nobody asked for one.

I took a shuttle bus to the Victoria Falls Hotel. We passed active minefields that were fenced off with skull-and-cross-bones signs that read, "Beware Minefields Danger." The mine-fields were between the road and the Zambezi River. Zambia was on the other side. The Falls Hotel looked like it had been frozen in time, a monument to the colonial past that seemed at odds with the changing character of the country. I recalled how we had always considered it too posh to stay at on our way to Chobe. I dined on the patio as the sun set and the night came on. I had Lion lager and a domestic white wine from Marondera. There were no imports. If you wanted something stiffer, you drank Mainstay, a spirit distilled from sugarcane that served as a substitute for gin or vodka, and which I suspected was closer to American moonshine.

The next morning I walked to the falls. The trolley line that used to carry guests between the hotel and the falls no longer ran, though the tracks were still there. The Zambezi was in full flood, surging over the falls in a deafening torrent that sent up such a dense cloud of mist from three hundred feet below that it was hard to see anything. I found Livingstone's statue and paused to think about the many times I'd visited it with my father. I walked around a bit. There was now a gate near the falls where admission was charged, but a short way off everything was still open. It was true jungle here, a rain forest on account of the continual soaking from the falls' spray.

At the hotel that evening, I ate in the dining room. As ever, jackets and ties were required. The waiters were black, in starched white uniforms, with white gloves and red fezzes. The food was good. I had crocodile tail, which reminded me of swordfish.

I wanted to see Botswana and Chobe—which was now part of a vast game reserve. I had planned to rent a car but learned that rentals were not permitted to cross the border. The day-long trip that used to take us through what had been North-ern Rhodesia and across the river to Kasungula by *makoro* was no longer necessary. There was now a road that followed the south bank of the Zambezi, so that you could now travel di-rectly to Botswana from Victoria Falls. It had been a dirt road at first, but it was paved during the war to prevent the planting of land mines along the route. Now it took just two hours to reach Kasane from Victoria Falls. I caught a minibus run by the Zimbabwe tourist board. I was the only passenger. A lively black man called Barnabas was the driver.

We rattled along the road to Kasungula, slowing at one point to allow a herd of sable antelope to cross the road. They then stood looking at us as we crawled past, their huge horns swept back against the sky. On we went. A blurry brown shape streaked across the road. "Lion," Barnabas said.

At Kasungula we encountered a sign that read, "Disease Control." We had to get out of the van, step on a wet mat, and re-turn to the vehicle. This was an effort to control foot and mouth disease. By nine in the morning, I was standing outside a hut in Kasane that rented four-wheel drive vehicles. An off-road car was a necessity in the soft Chobe sand, where getting stuck might invite the attention of elephants. Before it was a game reserve, I had made this trip alone many times, frequently at night, and was often surrounded by elephants as they made their way down to the river for their evening drink.

Kasane was no longer a sleepy little village but a town of thirty thousand, with several hotels. The Chobe River Hotel had changed since Charles Trevor's day. The hotel had expanded but was sadly rundown. I asked to stay in one of the original *rondavels* that Trevor had built. Then I had tea on the veranda overlooking the Chobe. The fast-flowing water was still high from the floods. While I sat there, a *makoro* came out of the reeds on the Namibian side and made its way across, carrying passengers who disembarked on reaching the Botswana side. So much for border control.

I was surprised to hear what had become of my boyhood friend Robert Holmes à Court. After Trevor was killed by bees, Holmes à Court emigrated to Australia, where he became a lawyer and then built a vast corporate empire that included wool production, transport, mining, and media. A feared corporate raider, he was the first Australian businessman to be worth more than a billion dollars and was now among the richest men in the world. A year after my visit to Chobe, Holmes à Court would die in his bed of a heart attack at the age of fifty-three. His mother had joined him in Perth, where he had a horse-breeding operation, after she sold the Chobe River Hotel. Against all odds, I met up with her a few years after my visit to Africa when I went to Perth to operate on a visiting English earl—he was the horse trainer to the queen of England—who was too sick to be transferred to America. This big world is, as the saying goes, sometimes a small place.

After tea, I set off for the game reserve. The road was rough enough to make it slow going. The bend that had been made to go around the carcass of the elephant shot by the district commissioner guarding Katharine Hepburn was still there, though after thirty years, no one knew why. The elephant population had soared after the game reserve was established, and the evidence of their presence was everywhere when I reached Chobe. Most of the big trees were gone, especially those that used to line the river, pushed over by the elephants to get to the juicy bark and branches on their upper limbs. There were elephant droppings everywhere, and plenty of signs of buffalo. But there were no elephants and buffalo around, as it was noon and getting hot.

I drove to Serondella, or rather, to the place where our cottage by that name used to be. Now there was a campsite named Serondella in its place. It was empty. A baboon was sitting on an overturned garbage can. I found Pop Lamont's grave near the riverbank, under the shade of one of the remaining trees. He'd been ordered out when the game reserve was established but had refused to leave. In the end they let him stay, perhaps because he had African children. Few in Kasane remembered or cared who he was. The early days of Chobe were mostly forgotten.

I had come to see elephants—some of which would surely be old acquaintances I'd known as a child. I drove along until I came across fresh tracks. I left the road and drove toward the river. Sure enough, there was an elephant herd moving through the scrub, headed to the water for a drink. One mother had a little baby. I backed the Land Rover into a clump of bushes to keep out of their way. Then several others I hadn't seen at first showed from where I'd come and started toward the Land Rover. I was downwind, so they had no idea I was there. Though they were not more than a few yards away, they didn't see me. The first group also turned in my direction then—and they had my scent. They halted twenty-five yards away, flapping their ears and raising their trunks to sniff the air. An elephant herd is ruled by the matriarch, and breeding herds with babies can be dangerous. I was concerned about some mothers in this herd who seemed agitated, but they eventually ambled away in front of me and into the water. One elderly female, who seemed to be in charge, stood her ground. She looked at me, waving her trunk and shuffling about, not knowing whether to come on or back off. I was now surrounded by elephants—one of which was nervous and blocking my way out. I started the engine and inched out toward her. She shuffled aside, allowing me to get back on the road.

I drove on to the lavish new Chobe Game Lodge, which was not far away. It was on the river just below Crocodile Island, perhaps two miles from where I had caught the black mamba. Cool and luxurious, the hotel had air-conditioning, several swimming pools, and splendid views of the river and the savanna stretching to the horizon beyond. It was full of rich Americans and Germans. Everyone was fitted out in tailored safari gear. This wasn't the Chobe I knew, which had been remote and wild. A few tame warthogs rooted around in the garden. Each morning and evening, the hotel took guests out to watch the animals.

After lunch I drove back into the bush again. There was no shortage of game, and by dark I'd seen my fill of animals—including two large herds of buffalo that must have numbered in the hundreds. After dark, trying to get out of the park before the gates closed, I ran into more elephants. One, frightened by the headlights, trumpeted menacingly. I switched off the lights, and after a few moments the elephant turned away. I was up at dawn and back into the reserve the next day. Some giraffes crossed the road in front of me. Later there were more buffalo, flanking me on either side of the road, chewing the grass and watching me with little interest.

I felt crosscurrents of emotion when it was time to leave. Chobe had changed, and I could never wholly revisit the world I'd known there. But many of the things that I remembered most fondly were as they always had been. The broad sweep of the river and the animals that roamed along it took me back to a childhood filled with such scenes. How remarkable it was that I'd grown up in an untamed place and had never once been harmed by animals—only to learn many years later that the most dangerous animal of all is my own species.

The bus picked me up on the road outside the car rental hut. There was a new driver, and this time I had company—a young English couple headed to Victoria Falls on their honeymoon, and a husband and wife in their seventies. The older man was organized. He had a tidy file with their passports and entry forms, which he filled out on the bus to speed their way through the border at Kasungula. But there was a problem clearing the checkpoint into Zimbabwe. On his way out, the man had declared all the currency he was carrying and had been required to leave a portion of his Zimbabwean notes at the checkpoint to retrieve on his return. Unfortunately, this money had been locked away in a safe, the key to which now could not be located. We were told the man who might have the key was probably coming on duty later that day—or possibly not, a classically African abundance of variables. The dilemma was resolved when the customs officials took up a collection to pay the man his money, which turned out to be a trivial sum. They would reimburse themselves when the key to the safe turned up, and everyone was congratulated on an ingenious solution to the problem. We climbed back into the bus and rattled down the road toward the falls.

....

I flew on to Lake Kariba, a reservoir on the Zambezi River that is the world's biggest man-made body of water. The dam was built when I was at Whitestone, flooding the Kariba Gorge. From the air, it was a breathtaking expanse of water that looked like it had always been there. When the dam was completed, thousands of animals were trapped on islands that continued to shrink as the waters rose. A rescue effort, called Operation Noah, was undertaken, during which everything from elephants and rhinos to snakes and lions were hauled off and relocated to dry land. I still remembered when that stretch of the Zambezi was a hot and humid valley buzzing with tsetse flies that carried sleeping sickness. Now it was water for as far as the eye could see.

I checked into the Caribbea Bay Hotel on the shore of Lake Kariba. Elegant and vaguely Spanish-looking, the hotel seemed out of place. I was surprised to discover that one of the other guests was the actor and director Clint Eastwood, who was staying there while making a movie, *White Hunter Black Heart*, a film based on the making of that earlier picture *The African Queen*. I was amused to see that among its amenities, the hotel rented windsurfers. You could pick them up right next to a sign warning, "Swim at Own Risk, Beware of Crocodiles." There are some huge crocs in Kariba, where the locals call them flat dogs. I heard stories about crocodiles climbing onto houseboats and pulling careless vacationers into the water. Supposedly, there was a six-foot-long croc along every hundred yards of the river. I was told that at least one person was eaten every week, which was not surprising, as I saw people washing themselves and their clothes in the river, standing in the water to their knees.

That night, in the bar, I ran into the son of someone who'd gone to Whitestone with me. His father was a farmer in the northern part of Rhodesia who was shot and killed on his farm during the war. Of the seventy white farmers in the area, only two survived the conflict.

The next morning I got a ride in the open back of a Land Rover to a small river town named Chirundu. We passed an elephant shortly after setting out, and then disturbed a huge male lion who had been lying by the side of the road. The lion grumpily trotted off into the bush. There were more elephants at the river. They were hunted here, and as a result were skittish and more ill-tempered than the elephants at Chobe. I got to Chirundu around noon. There were monkeys playing on the corrugated iron roofs of the village and climbing in the bougainvilleas. I bought food and supplies, rented a canoe, and loaded up for a four-day trip downriver to the Mana Pools, some sixty miles through the heart of one of the wildest parts of Africa.

I paddled mainly to steer, letting the current carry me. I reflected on my life, which in so many ways seemed to have come apart. I'd lost my childhood home to war and a warped sense of progress, while my career had paused ominously. The river reminded me of the journey we all take, starting out and moving with the flow, traveling into the unknown and staying alert to the dangers that might be anywhere along the way. Loss is in most ways unquantifiable, as is the sadness that accompanies it. I couldn't measure how I felt, and as I floated onward, I gave up trying.

Birds and animals were everywhere. There weren't many mosquitoes, but I took antimalaria medication. The weather was perfect, which would not have been the case in many other months of the year. In summer the heat would make the trip intolerable. Now in June the midwinter days were warm and pleasant, the nights cool. To my right was Zimbabwe, and on the left Zambia. I followed the border, drifting on an imaginary line. The Zimbabwe side was a game park. Rangers there fought an ongoing war with poachers, who crossed over from Zambia and shot rhinos with fully automatic AK-47s, taking the horns and leaving the carcasses. On average, one rhino was taken every day, and back then horns fetched $50,000, a fraction of what they're worth today. Poachers were shot on sight.

I stayed mainly to the Zimbabwean side, hoping to avoid trigger-happy Zambians, though there were more immediate threats. Hippos were everywhere. They like to wallow in shallow water. When alarmed, they head for the deep water. The secret is not to get between them and their refuge. When I came upon hippos out on a sandbar or standing in the shallows, I would head straight for them, banging on the side of the canoe to make them move. They'd career off into deeper water and I'd continue on. This wasn't necessarily safe, as hippos are not always predictable. At several places I could not find an easy route through the pods of hippo. My only choice then was to paddle hard and trust that if I passed over a hippo, it would not take an interest in me. When I was growing up, the father of one of my friends had gone on a canoe trip and been killed by a hippo.

Crocodiles have good hearing. They would slide off the sandbanks a hundred yards before I came to them, leaving big skid marks on the sand. Occasionally I surprised one, and with a splash and swirl, it would be gone.

At the end of each day, I looked for a sandbar in the middle of the river to make camp. The riverbank would be too dangerous on account of lions, as I didn't want to make a fire and invite the attention of either poachers or rangers. The odds of being shot without warning in such an encounter at night would not have been in my favor. I stayed close to my camp and tried to leave few tracks for the same reason. I was much less concerned about the animals. I knew lions would not swim the river to eat, and crocs don't generally feed at night. Still, I stayed alert to everything around me. I hadn't brought a gun, and it was good to feel the hairs on my neck prickle now and again.

I didn't have a tent, just a sleeping bag that I crawled into during the brief interlude between sundown and darkness. A brilliant spray of stars filled the night sky. I slept soundly, waking before dawn to a loud chorus of birds. After a cup of coffee, I was away again as the sun rose, lighting the mist that hung over the river. I let the current pull me on through the murk, listening to the sounds of hippos grunting contentedly somewhere ahead. Africa is nature's cathedral, and I found its wild congregation restorative. I was in the middle of nowhere—and at the center of everything.

After four idyllic days, I arrived at the Mana Pools Game Reserve camp and found it largely deserted. There was a canoe onshore with two large holes in it, the result of a hippo attack that had thrown the occupants into the river. They'd managed to escape. But the more disturbing news was that one of the park's rangers had been eaten by a lion the previous day. He had been tracking poachers and was sleeping under a tree that night. He didn't light a fire to avoid alerting the poachers, preferring to take his chances with the lions—a fatal decision, as it turned out. My life back in the United States seemed a long way away. But I knew it was there. A Land Rover was waiting to take me back to civilization. I climbed in and started thinking about how I would build a cardiac program in San Diego. I was ready to start again.

CHAPTER TWENTY-ONE
THE LONG VIEW

My team had got to UCSD ahead of me. When I arrived in July of 1989, Michael Kaye had already set up the offices of the *Journal of Heart and Lung Transplantation* and the International Registry for Heart and Lung Transplants. He was also working on our experimental laboratories. Jolene Kriett and Riyad Tarazi were there, as were the transplant coordinators, Ann Hayden and Becky Robert. Apart from Tarazi, the whole crew were from the Midwest. I was happy they were willing to pack up and come to California with me.

There were two hospitals associated with the university: the main university hospital in San Diego, called Hillcrest, and the Veterans Administration hospital. We operated at both. The work consisted of adult and congenital cardiac surgery and lung surgery. My chief operating room nurse from Minnesota, Carol Hamlin, used her vacation time to come to UCSD to get things organized and to help train our new operating room staff. When she left, she gave me a note that said, "Tough times never last, but tough people do."

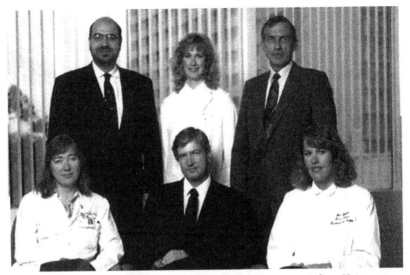

The team on arrival in San Diego (left to right) Front row: Jolene Kriett, me, and Ann Hayden. Back Row: Riyad Tarazi, Becky Robert, and Michael Kaye.

One day early on, when I returned to my office after operating, I found Moossa waiting to see me. He gave me a UCSD tie. In my three years in Minnesota, Najarian had never once come to my office. In fact, I don't think he ever visited the Heart and Lung Institute that I created.

The warm welcome at UCSD was nice, but I was eager to move the program forward. And I felt that because of what happened in Minnesota, I had no margin for error—there would be no second chance if I failed here. Although I trusted Kriett and Tarazi, at first I insisted on doing all of the difficult cases myself. This was a heavy workload, and it was challenging to navigate the resistance to my appointment. I still had to win over the people who'd threatened to leave if I came to San Diego.

The first was Ken Moser, whom I met when I was interviewing for the job. Moser was in charge of a strong pulmonary program that he'd founded in the early days of UCSD. He was an institution. His reputation rested largely on his work on thromboembolic disease, a condition in which high blood pressure in the lungs, or pulmonary hypertension, is caused by blood clots. I was also interested in this disease, because we were performing lung transplants for pulmonary hypertension. In fact, all of my first heart-and-lung transplants, which were among the first in the world, had been for this condition—which is a fairly common problem.

There are two types of pulmonary hypertension: one is caused by disease of the small pulmonary vessels, the cause of which is often unknown; the other is a disease of the larger vessels, usually the result of blood clots that travel from large veins in the body, pass through the heart, and become incorporated in a layer of scar tissue on the inner walls of the pulmonary arteries—where they obstruct the blood flow to the lungs. This "back pressure" eventually leads to heart failure. It also impedes the supply of oxygen to the body and causes shortness of breath.

Moser was an intimidating figure. He had trained one of my first mentors, Felix Eastcott. At Georgetown, Moser had persuaded Charles Hufnagel to remove clots from the lungs of a patient with chronic pulmonary hypertension way back in 1961. The operation, called a pulmonary thromboendarterectomy, or PTE for short, was a primitive and risky procedure then. The clots were removed while the heart was still beating. Heavy bleeding obscured the operating field so that it was hard for Hufnagel to see what he was doing.

When Moser moved to San Diego in 1968 as one of the founding members of the UCSD faculty, he convinced Nina Braunwald, a cardiac surgeon, to try the procedure. She did and it worked. In the intervening years, a handful of PTEs had been done by surgeons at UCSD, but without good success. When I arrived Pat Daily was the primary surgeon doing them at UCSD. Although a heart-and-lung transplant was one way to cure pulmonary hypertension, I was intrigued by the idea of coring out the pulmonary arteries with the PTE procedure. The fact that UCSD did this operation was one of the attractions of the job. I also thought I could do it better than they did—when I arrived, mortality in PTE surgeries was 20 percent.

After I replaced Daily as chief of cardiac surgery, he was still working at UCSD and at Sharp. I wanted to end this dual enterprise, which was one of the main reasons Moossa had hired me. Daily lobbied hard to stay, doing his best to convince his colleagues at UCSD that he was indispensable. Ken Moser was a strong Daily ally, which was why he had been so opposed to my appointment. Moser didn't think that anyone but Daily could do the PTE operation. Moser's threat to resign was still on the table.

I'd only been in town a short time when Moossa invited Daily and me to dinner at his favorite haunt, the Fairbanks Country Club. The purpose was to discuss how we could work together at UCSD—though I had a hunch that wasn't really what Moossa was hoping for. Daily arrived all swagger, ready for a fight.

Daily told Moossa that he would leave the university if he was not allowed to do all the children and all the pulmonary thromboendarterectomies while he continued to work at Sharp. In plain language, he wanted nothing to change—and he demanded a written contract to that effect. This would have meant that Daily kept the bulk of the cardiac surgery. This was unacceptable, but I knew that Daily had the backing of many of the cardiologists at the university in addition to Ken Moser and the pulmonary group. I had to decide on the spot how hard to fight.

I told Moossa I could not agree to Daily's demand, and that if Moossa accepted Daily's ultimatum, it would be me who left. Moossa stared at me. I didn't want to find myself on the street again. But I also didn't want my first major decision at UCSD to be the wrong one. Moossa turned to Daily.

"Well, Pat," he said calmly, "I have to side with Stuart."

Daily pushed his chair back, got up from the table without saying a word, and walked out. Moossa and I were left looking at each other over Daily's half-eaten dinner. I apologized for putting him in a difficult position.

"On the contrary, Stuart," he said, "if you had not said that, I would have known I had the wrong man for the job."

Daily kept his word and never set foot in the university hospital again. I went to see Moser the next day to tell him that from now on pulmonary hypertension cases were university patients and would be operated on by university faculty. Daily, I said, was no longer on the faculty.

Moser, who must have already heard this from Daily, didn't flinch. "Well, Stuart," he said, "you've never done a pulmonary thromboendarterectomy."

I said that was true, but that I'd done thousands of open-heart operations and had pioneered new techniques. I was confident I could do the PTE and do it better than Daily. Moser was skeptical. So I proposed a deal. For six months, Moser could send half the pulmonary patients to Daily—on the condition that he sent the other half to me. At the end of that time, he would be free to send the patients to whichever surgeon he felt was better.

Moser agreed. And at the end of six months, he started sending all of the patients to me.

That was when Daily made a big mistake. He stormed into Moser's office, banged on the desk, and insisted that the fifty-fifty sharing arrangement be continued. Nobody threatened Ken Moser. He ordered Daily out of his office and never spoke to him again. Daily subsequently advertised his pulmonary thromboendarterectomy program at Sharp Hospital. But it failed after a handful of cases and was discontinued.

With Daily gone, I could build the thromboendarterectomy program. I modified the technique and developed new instruments for the operation, which can take all day. The objective is to remove the layer of clot from inside the artery by peeling it from the artery wall with a fine blade. It is delicate work: the artery wall is only as thick as the page on which you're reading this. Once you establish the plane between the clot and the artery wall, you follow it, working ever deeper until you get it all out. This has to be done under intense magnification, and you can't have any blood in the operating field. That means the heart can't be beating and you can't have the heart-lung machine pumping. You have to shut it all down and drain all the blood from the patient. If you did only that, you would have at most a few minutes to work before you caused brain damage.

So we used John Lewis's old method: hypothermia. We put the patient on bypass and then use the heart-lung machine to cool the patient. Then we drain all the blood and hold it in the heart-lung machine while we work. With no blood supply to the brain, or to any of the other organs, you still only have twenty minutes to work, even under hypothermia. So, after twenty minutes, we turn the heart-lung machine back on. After ten minutes we do it all again, draining the blood and continuing the surgery for another twenty minutes. And so on, until we are done and the patient is warmed again.

This raises an interesting question. What is the status of the patient during the operating phase of the procedure? There is no heartbeat, no blood flow. Brain activity is flatlined. Is the patient dead? I don't think anyone can answer that. But I do know one thing: after thousands of surgeries during which patients have hovered in this netherworld, none of them has ever awakened and said they saw a bright light, or the pearly gates, or the face of God himself. Not one. If those patients are on the "other side" while we operate, it is a black void.

We saw a dramatic improvement in PTE outcomes right away. We had been doing one or two PTE cases a month. Now that jumped to two or three a week. By 1998, I had done more than a thousand of these cases, and in 2003 I presented the results of the first fifteen hundred cases at the annual Society of Thoracic Surgeons meeting. At the time, hardly anyone else was doing the operation. Just as with the paper that I had presented to the same conference on combined heart-and-lung transplantation years earlier, this one was named the most significant of the meeting. The honor was especially rewarding, because it was the only time it had been given twice to the same person.

The society had invited my old Stanford colleague Chris McGregor, now from the Mayo Clinic, to discuss the paper. He congratulated me for developing the "world's leading pulmonary endarterectomy practice," and for the team approach we'd taken at UCSD in managing "this demanding disease." McGregor also pointed to the value of the research efforts in the lab that supported our clinical practice. I was gratified that it was understood that a surgical procedure is of limited value if only one person can do it. Training other members of my team to do the PTE—and welcoming surgical teams from all over the world to train with us—was essential.

The PTE program at UCSD remains the best in the world. Although it is probably the most difficult of all surgical procedures—it lasts all day and is almost always done on desperately sick patients—our success rate is comparable to that of regular open-heart surgeries, with a mortality rate of only about 2 percent. That includes patients who arrive by helicopters and are being kept alive on ventilators.

....

One day early in my tenure at UCSD, just after I'd done the first heart transplant ever performed at the university, the chief cardiologist told me about a patient with heart disease. He had narrowing of the aortic valve and also severe coronary disease. But the cardiologist was hesitant to refer him for surgery, as the patient was in his eighties. Not only that, he was a person of considerable influence at UCSD. An unsuccessful outcome would not be good for our program. I told the cardiologist I didn't care who it was. Everyone gets the same level of care. Yes, a patient that old was a high-risk candidate for surgery, but without it he would die.

This elderly patient turned out to be Roger Revelle, a founder of UCSD and a man with an international reputation. The first college at UCSD was named for him. Revelle had also been head of the Scripps Institute of Oceanography and had done pioneering work on the warming of the oceans. He coined the term *the greenhouse effect*. Revelle was a friend of the former president Ronald Reagan. Just as Stan had been among my most important early cases at Minnesota, an adverse outcome for Revelle could destroy my career at UCSD. He went on the schedule.

I was in the OR when the cardiologist came in late one afternoon to tell me he had just performed a heart catheterization on Revelle. He said the patient's condition was "a little rocky." Asking one of my colleagues to finish up, I left the operating room and went to see him. Revelle was pale and sweating, clammy to the touch, and asleep with labored breathing. His blood pressure was dangerously low. The cardiologist looked grim and suggested that perhaps it was too late for surgery.

I ordered Revelle straight to the operating room.

Once he was on the heart-lung machine, I went to work, replacing his aortic valve and performing bypasses for all three coronary arteries. The phone in the OR rang. It was the president of the university, asking me to phone him with a report on Revelle's condition as soon as the operation was over, regardless of the time. I called him back just after midnight to say that Revelle had come through the operation and was recovering.

The next day there was a long story in the newspaper about Revelle and also our first heart transplant. I was worried about how the coverage would be, since the newspapers in San Diego had picked up on some of the controversy surrounding my hiring. Their initial reporting focused on the salaries members of my team were getting, and on the accusations that had followed me from Minnesota. But I needn't have worried. I was no longer described as a "controversial" surgeon, but a "pioneering" one. That felt like a win.

Bill Baxt, the hospital chief of staff, sent me a memo saying, "Congratulations, we are proud to have you here at UCSD." Moossa, unlike Najarian, who took credit for every success we had, happily acknowledged the progress of the cardiac unit at every step. After we did Southern California's first combined heart-and-lung transplant the next month, the dean sent over a dozen heart-shaped balloons with a message saying, "The university is proud of you."

....

I had been at UCSD for about a year when one of the cardiologists came to me with an angiogram that showed a patient in severe difficulty. The heart was barely beating, and the coronary vasculature, the blood supply to the heart, was badly compromised. This patient's left coronary tree, which supplied blood to the main pumping chamber of the heart, was totally blocked. This condition is rare, because a total blockage in this location is almost always fatal. The patient had survived because he was fortunate enough to have an additional blood supply from the right coronary artery, though it, too, was severely diseased. I told the cardiologist that I thought the patient needed a heart transplant.

"The patient is Kenneth Moser," he said.

I was crushed. Ken was not a candidate for a heart transplant. We were not doing people his age at the time. And I doubted he'd submit to the procedure anyway. But without some kind of surgical intervention, Moser would soon be dead. The alternative to a transplant was a risky operation in which some of the dead heart muscle would be cut out in conjunction with a coronary artery bypass.

I talked it over with Moser. He could have asked any heart surgeon in the world to do it. He asked me.

The operation went well. Moser recovered and went back to work. A few weeks later, I received a call from his secretary. "I hope I'm not being disloyal," she said nervously, "but Dr. Moser has started smoking again, and I think you ought to speak to him about it."

This was hard to believe. The man in charge of a renowned pulmonary department, who had been the president of the most important pulmonary medical society, the American College of Chest Physicians, smoked! And he continued to smoke after having heart problems that almost killed him. I walked over to his office and sat down. Ken was happy to see me and asked what was on my mind.

"Ken," I said, "I've come here as your friend, as a colleague, and as your surgeon."

"Yes?" he said.

"I've come to talk about your smoking," I said.

"Stuart, is there anything else you want to talk about?"

"No, Ken," I said, "that's it."

He pointed the way out of his office and said, "There's the door." I was beaten.

More than a year later, Bill Auger, one of Moser's bright young assistants, showed me a chest X-ray with a large mass visible, a lung cancer. It was Ken's X-ray. Again, we operated, this time removing part of his lung. He continued to smoke. After he had recovered from his lung operation, I would see him walking toward his car in in the evenings, wheeling a bottle of oxygen with his left hand and holding a cigarette in his right. Ken died on June 9, 1997, a little more than seven years after we first worked together. He was sixty-eight, not young certainly, but not old, either.

By the time Moser died, we had done a total of 855 PTE operations and were by far the leading PTE program in the world. I worried that Ken's death, which had affected me deeply, would also have an impact on our practice. He had been our primary referring pulmonologist, bringing us a steady flow of patients, including many from other countries. I should not have worried. Like all great leaders, Ken had trained and gathered around him a group of talented individuals who were up to the task of carrying on. Our team has now done more than four thousand of these operations.

....

Being a surgeon does not make you immune to ordinary human emotions. I was home one evening around Christmas—a rarity for me—when the phone rang. A surgeon who was a close friend was on the line. He was out of breath. He told me his mother, who was visiting from Europe, had suffered a cardiac arrest. He was administering CPR on his kitchen floor. I asked him if he'd called 911.

"No, boss," he said. "I'm calling you."

It's funny how the mind works in a moment like that, how a brilliant guy like my friend wasn't thinking straight, even though he'd handled a situation like this many times. When it's family, it's different. I told him to hang up and call 911 and then call me back after he did. He called back in a bit and said they were in an ambulance headed to Scripps Memorial, which was not our hospital but was the closest. I said I'd meet him at the emergency room. The surgeon and his mother got there before I did.

When I came in, the staff looked ashen. They pointed me to a room. When I went in, several doctors and nurses were standing there in shock. My friend had picked up a scalpel and opened his mother's chest in a desperate attempt to save her. He was doing direct heart massage with his bare hand. I watched for a few minutes, and it was plain that it was hopeless. I walked over and pulled his bloody hand from his mother's chest and held him by the shoulders.

"You've got to stop now," I said. "Your mother is dead."

We went back to his apartment, where I spent the night with him, talking, trying to help him come to terms with his mother's sudden death. We were having a brandy when he realized he had to call his father, who was in Europe.

"What should I tell him?" he asked.

"Don't tell him your mother has died," I said. "He'll never be able to get on an airplane if you do. Tell him that she's had a heart attack and is in the hospital and that he should come at once." I knew the long plane ride from Europe would give him time to prepare for the worst.

....

Most of the time, a surgeon's life is one of daily rewards. I had wanted to fix people when I was young and dreaming of becoming a surgeon. In heart and lung surgery, you do more than just fix people—you restore them to a life they've been forced to stop living. They're not fixed. They're transformed.

One day I left the operating room around noon and walked to my office. My secretary told me that someone was waiting inside to see me. When I went in, I found a healthy-looking man accompanied by his son seated on my sofa.

"You won't remember me," the man said as he stood up to shake hands. "I'm Joe."

I remembered him perfectly. When I operated on Joe in 1982, he was one of the world's first heart-and-lung transplants. He had called me earlier that year. He was my age at the time, thirty-four, and had a wife and a five-year-old son. Joe had been told he had only a few months to live. He said he would give anything, pay any price, to live long enough to see his son go to college. He had read about some of our early heart-and-lung transplants in the newspapers and wondered if I could help. He asked about our experience with the operation. I told him we had a lot of experience in monkeys, but not much as yet in humans. He laughed, and said, "Well, I really don't have much choice, do I?"

I agreed that he didn't and asked him to come see us.

I spent a lot of time with Joe when he got to Stanford. He'd come with his wife and son. After careful consideration, we decided to put him on the list. The time came when we had a suitable donor and did the transplant. It was in the night, as usual. Everything went smoothly. After the operation, Joe was in an isolation room that I passed by every day on my way to the OR. I'd pause to look through the big glass doors. Almost without fail, Joe's son, dressed in a blue sterile gown, with gloves on and wearing a surgical mask that was too big for him, was in bed with him. At the time I thought that if I never did another thing worthwhile, this would be accomplishment enough.

Joe left the hospital and went back to his life. Years passed. I moved to Minnesota and then back to California. Now, here he was sitting in my office with his grown son. I told Joe I remembered everything about him and his operation, including the date and even what his temperature was on his tenth postoperative day. He laughed.

"Well, you do remember me," he said. "I'm here because I'm bringing my son to UCSD to look at the college."

So, he'd made it, lived to see the day his son would go to college. He looked fit and happy. Joe was then the longest-living combined heart-and-lung transplant recipient in the world—and surely among the luckiest fathers who ever lived.

....

Although conventional heart surgery was going to be the main part of our practice in the new program at UCSD, I wanted to start our transplant programs immediately. Heart transplantation had not yet been done at the university. Double-lung and single-lung transplantation had never been done in Southern California. Ideally, a transplant program is a joint effort between the surgeons and the physicians—pulmonologists for lung transplantation and cardiologists for heart transplantation. Cecilia Smith, a university pulmonologist, was eager to be involved. But we were not so lucky with heart transplantation. We could not generate any enthusiasm from the cardiologists. No one wanted to be included. When we were promised help, Pat Daily's old friend, the chief of cardiology, was appointed chairman of the search committee to recruit a cardiologist to work with the transplant program. Every person I suggested for the post apparently had a defect of which I was unaware. The committee finally disbanded without interviewing a single candidate. I decided to start the program on my own, without any input from cardiology.

This worked fine. It was like Minnesota all over again. We promoted the program. I gave talks at all the neighboring hospitals. My group took the referrals of patients in end-stage heart failure and assessed the candidates. After a slow start, we soon had a number of good candidates for the operation. Within six months of my arrival in San Diego, we were ready to go ahead.

We did the medical workups, found money or insurance to cover the cost, did the operations and all the postoperative care, including immunosuppression and the long-term follow-up. We continued to work this way for three years. We became a Medicare-approved center of excellence after two years and started getting paid by the government for transplants. Our results were exceptional, the best in the US and likely the entire world. Of our first fifty transplant patients, only one did not make it.

Our first heart transplant was done in February 1990 on a Sunday afternoon. Moossa came into the operating room "to lend moral support," he said. I also heard from Roger Revelle, who was still in the hospital recovering from his surgery. He and his wife, Ellen, who was part of the Scripps family, offered to help with whatever hospital bills the patient could not cover. The operation went well, and the patient was soon discharged. A month later, we did the first combined heart-and-lung transplant at UCSD. Renee Williams, a nurse, had pulmonary hypertension from a congenital heart defect. It wasn't possible to simply close the hole in her heart now, because her lungs had become irreversibly damaged. The operation took place during the night on March 13, 1990. It was almost four years since I had done the Midwest's first heart-and-lung transplant. That patient is still doing well more than thirty years later, the longest-living lung transplant in the world.

In the beginning, not everyone was clear about who would benefit from a heart transplant. I remember getting a call from a nearby hospital about a woman they believed needed one. I'd had a long day in the operating room but walked over to see her in the evening. The patient was a wizened, elderly black woman. She must have been at least eighty. She was sitting up in bed with a skullcap on. What little hair showed beneath it was snowy white. Not only was she well past the age when we would consider doing a transplant, her chart indicated that she was also in the end stages of cirrhosis from alcohol abuse. But I thought that since I'd come over and introduced myself, I should spend a little time explaining what we did. It soon became apparent that no one had brought up the idea of a transplant with her. Which was just as well.

"Nobody's cutting on me," she said. "Don't want no knife."

I couldn't disagree with that. Realizing she would not be disappointed at not getting a transplant, I went on and explained the procedure to her so she could feel confident in turning it down. She listened patiently. I wasn't sure she understood what I was talking about. But she did—perfectly.

"So let me get this right," she said, "You goin' to take out my ticker box and replace it with someone else's ticker box? From someone that's died?"

"That's right," I said.

"Well," she said, poking me in the chest with a bony finger, "tell me this, sonny boy. If it couldn't keep them alive, how's it going to keep me alive?"

I told her she had an excellent point.

The transplant programs at UCSD continued to grow. In early 1990, we did four transplants in one day—a heart in the early hours of one morning, and then two lungs and a heart simultaneously in the evening, with three operating rooms running at the same time. In between I did three other heart operations. Within a year of our arrival in San Diego, my team had done seventeen lung transplants, and after the first three years, more than one hundred heart, lung, or heart-and-lung transplants with well over a 90 percent survival rate at one year. These patients included the first lung-only transplants in California, as Stanford was still only doing combined heart-and-lung operations. We did the first double-lung transplant the next year, in January 1991. The patient had cystic fibrosis, did well, and was soon out of the hospital.

I always thought the cystic fibrosis patients were special. A lifetime of struggling to breathe had made them fighters, and they were tremendously grateful for any help that we could give them. I remember one twenty-one-year-old college student named Maria. She came to us desperately ill and wasting away. She weighed only eighty pounds when we did her double-lung transplant. I went to see her before she went home, two weeks after the surgery.

"Dr. Jamieson, I feel great!" she said.

I told her I was happy to hear it.

"No," she said, "I feel *great*."

Again, I said I was delighted.

"No," she said, "you're not hearing me. For twenty-one years, I have felt sick. I have never felt well. And now, for the very first time in my life, I feel well. I feel normal. I feel great! You don't know what you do."

Maria's mother, who was sitting by the bed, assured her that we knew. Maybe so, but sometimes it helped when we were reminded. I listened as Maria told me how she would now be able to go to sleep at night without hearing herself wheezing and gurgling, and not be afraid that she'd wake up in the night struggling for air. She was thrilled that she'd be able to get on an airplane, see places like Rome or Paris. Maria said she had something that I realized most of us take for granted: a future.

A few days after that, I went fishing, though I still carried my beeper. Except for the three months I'd spent in Africa, I had been continuously on call for more than twelve years. Tomorrow was Easter Sunday. When I returned home in the evening, a basket of flowers and an Easter card were waiting for me. "Thank you for our miracle," the card read. It was signed by Maria and her family.

In 1992 we did something new. Sam, a young boy with cystic fibrosis, was dying. We couldn't find a donor because of his small size. He was in the end stages of lung failure. At best he had two weeks to live. I lay awake at night thinking about what we could do to save his life. I had an idea, but it was something that had never been attempted, and it was risky. I told Sam's parents that if we took a part of each of their lungs, we could replace Sam's lungs entirely. They agreed without hesitation. We tested their lung functions, and both were good. They could get by just fine with one lobe of their lungs removed. The size and tissue match of each parent was suitable for Sam.

But I still wasn't sure it was a good idea. The main problem for me was the issue of informed consent. Any parent would give his or her own life for their child. How objective could they be if I was only asking them to give up a piece of their lungs? What finally convinced me to go ahead was that I believed the risks to the parents were minimal—and more than justified if Sam could live. Not all of my colleagues were as confident. One of them told me I would go down in history as the first surgeon to have a 300 percent mortality for one operation by killing the child and both parents. I was reminded of how Walt Lillehei had been warned he'd have a 200 percent mortality in his first cross-circulation operation. I told my friend that I was sure the operation could be done safely, but I pointed out that a 300 percent mortality in one operation had happened before.

Robert Liston, a pioneering Scottish surgeon born in 1794, practiced in the days before anesthesia and antibiotics. Survival of surgical patients then depended on speed. The faster the surgery, the less the bleeding and pain, and the smaller the opportunity for the wound to become infected. Nobody understood the concept of sterility then. Liston operated in a frock coat and waterproof boots. He was, to be sure, fast. To save time after making the incision, he would hold the knife between his teeth if he had to then saw through bone. On one occasion, he amputated a patient's leg in two and a half minutes, but in his haste his knife also amputated the patient's testicles. In the operation that achieved 300 percent mortality, he amputated the leg of a patient who died afterward from a gangrenous wound infection. Liston's knife also slashed through the coat tails of a distinguished spectator, who, terrified, had a heart attack and died. The flashing blade also amputated the fingers of his young assistant, who died afterward from infection.

I knew I would do better than Liston.

We worked in three operating rooms and with three teams. We removed part of the father's right lung and used it to replace Sam's entire right lung, and then part of the mother's left lung to replace Sam's entire left lung. The operation went exactly as planned—everyone survived. But Sam had a difficult postoperative course, in part because each lung rejected at a different rate. It was hard to differentiate between rejection and infection. But Sam gradually improved and ultimately left the hospital with a new lease on life. After a few more of these "living-related" transplants, I stopped doing them, still grappling with the risk to the parent donors. I was mindful of the injunction that is central to the practice of medicine: first, do no harm. I was not satisfied that we could always avoid harming a parent with what was, after all, not a minor procedure but major surgery.

In early 1994, I got a call from a Dr. Janssen, who wanted to consult with me about a baby with an atrial septal defect, a hole in the entrance chamber of the heart. Janssen wanted to know when it should be closed. I asked him how old the infant was and how much it weighed. He said two months and fifty pounds.

"Fifty pounds?" I was incredulous.

"Yes," he said. "That's very small for a baby orangutan."

Janssen had neglected to say that he was the head veterinarian at the San Diego Zoo. Once I understood, he asked if we could help.

I went to the zoo and found that they had a state-of-the-art operating room. We tested the orangutan family to see which one would be a suitable blood donor, and later in the summer the whole team went over to the zoo on a Saturday morning to do open-heart surgery on the little ape. It was almost like operating on a human child, except for the heavy chest muscles needed for swinging through the trees, and a large pouch over the airway for the throaty calls orangutans make. The surgery was filmed by a camera crew from the zoo. During the operation we received a call that an infant donor heart was available. We had a baby waiting for a transplant back at UCSD.

We finished the orangutan by noon and went immediately back to the university hospital, where we transplanted the baby—San Diego's first heart transplant in an infant. Later that month we did the first lung transplant in a child.

Neither operation attracted as much attention as the one on the ape. The day after doing it, I left for Costa Rica, where I was giving a talk at a conference. I arrived in the evening tired, sat down in my room, put my feet up, and turned on the television to catch up on the day's news. And right there on CNN I saw myself operating on the orangutan. *Well*, I thought, *I am famous at last.*

The orangutan grew up. Her name is Karen, and she now has offspring of her own. There's a plaque at the orangutan exhibit saying that Karen was the first of her endangered species to have open-heart surgery and acknowledging Dr. Jolene Kriett and me for doing the procedure. Naturally we published details of the operation—in the *Journal of Zoological and Wildlife Medicine.*

In 1991, we did a lung transplant on a man in his sixties, then the world's oldest recipient. Manuel Mateos Cándano came from old family in Mexico City, where he was a well-known physician, local mayor, and head of the medical society. He was also a lifelong smoker. By his late fifties, emphysema had forced him to leave the high altitude and smog of Mexico City, where the air pollution was so dense that birds sometimes fell from the sky. He moved first to Acapulco, at sea level, where it was easier to breathe. Cándano was lonely there. He could see no future for himself and often thought of ending it all. Cándano moved again, this time to Tijuana to be closer to medical care in the US. That's when an old friend told him about the lung transplant program at UCSD.

Manuel came to my office in a wheelchair and on oxygen. He was pale and gasping for every breath, struggling to stay alive from one moment to the next. I was impressed by his determination and will to live. He was the oldest patient we had accepted, but I said we'd put him on our list. That meant Cándano had to begin active rehabilitation therapy, to try to get his strength back for the operation to come. One day I saw him in the clinic for his eleven a.m. appointment. He told me he'd gotten up at five. When I asked him why so early, he explained that he needed that much time to get ready. Manuel said buttoning one button on his shirt took five minutes, brushing his teeth twenty. He said that back home he was tethered to an oxygen tank with fifty feet of tubing—"like a goat to a post," he said. Manuel said there were parts of his house he had never seen. I realized then how much a transplant would change his life.

Months passed. And then we got a call about a donor with good lungs that would be the right fit for Manuel and another patient we had waiting. We decided to use one lung for Manuel and the other for the other patient. We did the operations simultaneously—Jolene did one and I did the other. Both went well. We finished around five a.m., ready to begin yet another full day of surgery.

Manuel recovered. He threw away his oxygen equipment and went back to Mexico City, a place he never thought he would see again. He returned to his surgical practice with his son as his partner.

Some years later, I went to Mexico City to give a talk. I met Manuel for lunch. He looked terrific. He invited me to spend a couple of days with him at his ranch. It was a pretty place, nestled in a valley with a river running through it, about two hours north of Mexico City. Butterflies migrate there every year. Manuel kept horses and could ride again. Early one morning, as dawn broke, I got up to enjoy the sunrise. To my surprise Manuel was already up, standing on the porch, looking across the valley to the hills on the other side. I asked what he was doing. "I am looking at my lung," he said. "I sold that land over there, on the other side of the river, to pay for my lung transplant. That is my new life over there, my lung."

....

Heart transplantation has become almost routine, and lung transplantation is now commonly performed by many groups around the world. It is sometimes difficult to remember the difficulties we encountered in those early days, when we were doing things that many thought were impossible. Experimental work with cyclosporin in our lab at Stanford moved heart transplantation into a new phase, opened the door to lung transplantation, and led us to discover other antirejection drugs. I was fortunate to have been part of that effort.

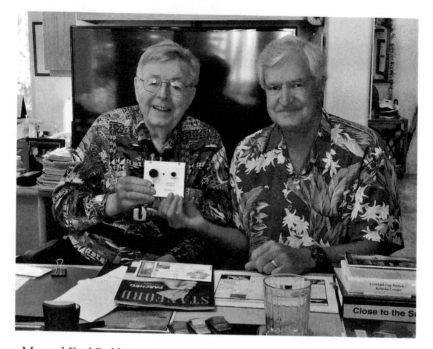

Me and Earl Bakken, inventor of the first transistorized pacemaker and founder of Medtronic, at his home in Hawaii. We are holding the first pacemaker—used in a child in 1957. An early draft of Close to the Sun *is on his desk.*

What has remained vivid to me are the people we were able to save when they seemed beyond help. The longest-surviving heart, lung, and heart-and-lung transplant patients in the world are people I operated on. Many of them are alive today because we pushed back the limitations on what we could do and for whom we could do it. Over time, transplant patients got older. And younger. And our progress is far from over. Today we perform coronary bypass operations without using the heart-lung machine. We can do complex heart surgeries through small incisions, or replace a heart valve through a catheter that requires no incision at all. In the future we'll use robots that will allow us to operate remotely—doing heart surgery anywhere in the world without leaving our home hospital. One day we'll use stem cells to regenerate heart tissue damaged by a heart attack, and we'll make whole new organs with 3-D printers. As we keep learning, anything really is possible.

All of this has taken place in a field that did not exist when I was born. The earliest pioneers of open-heart surgery were my mentors and eventually my friends. I have been lucky to be part of something important, to have had a hand in advancing the surgical procedures that have helped so many. I was wise to fly close to the sun.

I could write a book about my now thirty years at UCSD. But that is another story for another time. In 2011, twenty-two years after I came to San Diego with a promise to build it, the $250 million Cardiovascular Center opened. Mike Kaye and Jolene Kriett have retired. Riyad Tarazi left to head a heart program in Kuwait. Of our original group at UCSD, only I am still there. Most of my time is spent training the next generation of heart surgeons. I have a fancy title—distinguished professor of surgery and dean for cardiovascular affairs—and I recently traveled to Cape Town to receive a Living Legend award from the World Society of Cardiovascular and Thoracic Surgeons. These honors make me wonder if I am getting old, though being a living legend is preferable to the alternative.

When I came to UCSD, 250 open heart surgeries a year were being done. I was brought here to build the program. We now do twenty-five hundred heart surgeries a year, making us one of the busiest heart centers in the world. The team consists mainly of people I have trained.

I still operate, but not as much as before. I have now been involved in more than forty thousand heart surgeries, extending the lives of enough patients to populate a small city. Surgeons I have trained—and who will themselves train their successors—have saved many thousands more lives. My work is alive.

So am I. Now I contemplate the future and what it holds. I can do whatever I want. I hear there is land for sale in Chobe, and Africa still lives in my blood. I wouldn't mind renewing my friendship with the elephants. A few of the old ones might remember me.

POSTSCRIPT

Richard Atkinson
Richard Chatham Atkinson earned his bachelor's degree at the University of Chicago and a PhD in experimental psychology and mathematics at Indiana University. Atkinson joined the faculty at Stanford University in 1956, where he was professor of psychology from 1956 to 1975. He was then nominated by President Jimmy Carter to be the director of the National Science Foundation, a position he served in from 1975 to 1980. He was then appointed chancellor of the University of California, San Diego, and in October 1995 was made the University of California's seventeenth president. He turned eighty-nine in March 2018.

Leonard Bailey
Leonard Lee Bailey is surgeon in chief at Loma Linda University Children's Hospital. He placed the heart of a baboon into the chest of "Baby Fae," an infant born with a severe heart defect known as hypoplastic left heart syndrome, on October 26,

---

* *Biographical information has been supplied to the author by all respective parties.*

1984. Baby Fae only lived twenty-one days before she died, but the operation marked the beginning of infant heart transplants, although baboon hearts were not used again. Bailey continued to pioneer infant heart transplantation. "Baby Moses," transplanted by Bailey in 1985, is the oldest living infant heart-transplant recipient.

Earl Bakken

Earl E. Bakken was an American engineer, businessman and philanthropist. He founded Medtronic, where he developed the first external, battery-operated, transistorized, wearable artificial pacemaker in 1957. Bakken had a long-held fascination with electricity and electronics. A self-described "nerd," Bakken designed a rudimentary electroshock weapon in school to fend off bullies. After earning a bachelor of science in electrical engineering in 1948, he studied electrical engineering with a minor in mathematics at the University of Minnesota Graduate School. Post-World War II hospitals were just starting to employ electronic equipment but did not have staff to maintain and repair them. With his brother-in-law, Palmer Hermundslie, he formed Medtronic (the combination of "medical" and "electronic") in a small garage, primarily working with the University of Minnesota hospital.

Over the next several years, Bakken and Medtronic worked with other doctors to develop fully implantable pacemakers, but they also veered toward bankruptcy. He borrowed money that kept Medtronic going.

Bakken retired from Medtronic in 1989 and moved to a nine-acre estate in the Kona District of Hawaii. In 1996 he helped to dedicate the North Hawaii Community Hospital and has been active there ever since, working to combine Eastern and Western approaches to medicine to develop a more holistic approach to health care. Bakken died on October 21, 2018 at the age of ninety-four.

Christiaan Barnard

Christiaan Neethling Barnard matriculated from Beaufort West High School in South Africa in 1940 and studied medicine at the University of Cape Town, graduating in 1945. He did his internship and residency at the Groote Schuur Hospital in Cape Town. In 1956, he received a two-year scholarship, which he used for postgraduate training in cardiothoracic surgery at the University of Minnesota, under Walt Lillehei. Norman Shumway and Matt Paneth were there at the same time. Upon returning to South Africa in 1958, Barnard was appointed cardiothoracic surgeon at the Groote Schuur Hospital and did the first human-to-human heart transplant there in December 1967. He retired in 1983. Barnard became obsessed with staving off old age, and his reputation suffered when he promoted *Glycel*, an expensive "antiaging" skin cream, whose approval was soon withdrawn by the US Food and Drug Administration. He also spent time as a research adviser to the Clinique la Prairie, in Switzerland, where controversial "rejuvenation therapy" was practiced. He died on September 2, 2001, while on holiday in Cyprus at the age of seventy-eight, apparently from an asthma attack.

Denton Cooley

Denton Arthur Cooley graduated in 1941 from the University of Texas at Austin and began his medical education at the University of Texas Medical Branch in Galveston. He completed his medical degree and his surgical training at the Johns Hopkins School of Medicine in Baltimore, Maryland, where he also did his internship. At Johns Hopkins, he worked with Alfred Blalock and assisted in the first "blue baby" procedure to correct an infant's congenital heart defect. He completed his residency at Johns Hopkins and remained there as an instructor in surgery. In 1950 he went to London to work with Lord Russell Brock at the Brompton Hospital. After London he moved to Houston, Texas, where he worked with Michael E. DeBakey at the Baylor College of Medicine. In 1960, Cooley moved his practice to St. Luke's Episcopal Hospital while continuing to teach at Baylor. In 1962 he founded the Texas Heart Institute with private funds and, following a dispute with DeBakey, resigned his position at Baylor in 1969. He was the first heart surgeon to implant an artificial heart in a man, Haskell Karp, who lived for sixty-five hours. Cooley authored or coauthored more than fourteen hundred scientific articles and twelve books. He was awarded the Presidential Medal of Freedom by Ronald Reagan in 1984. Dr. Cooley died on November 18, 2016, aged ninety-six.

Pat Daily

Patrick Daily obtained a bachelor's degree in biology from the University of Oklahoma and his medical degree from the University of Chicago in 1962. He did a cardiovascular surgery residency at Stanford University and then went to San Diego in 1973. He worked at UCSD and also at Sharp Memorial Hospital but moved to Sharp exclusively in 1989. In his midsixties he developed Alzheimer's disease, and he died on April 25, 2008, aged seventy-one.

Terence English

Sir Terence English was born in South Africa and initially became a mining engineer. He later decided to study medicine and did some of his early training under Matt Paneth at the Brompton Hospital. He was consultant cardiothoracic surgeon at Papworth Hospital and Addenbrooke's Hospital, Cambridge, from 1973 to 1995. He performed Britain's first successful heart transplant in August 1979, after which Papworth became one of the leading heart and lung transplant centers in Europe. He was president of the Royal College of Surgeons from 1989 to

1992; master of St. Catharine's College, Cambridge, from 1993 to 2000; and president of the British Medical Association from 1995 to 1996. He was knighted in 1991. English received the Lifetime Achievement Award from the Society for Cardiothoracic Surgery in Great Britain and Ireland in 2009, and the Lifetime Achievement Award from the International Society for Heart and Lung Transplantation in 2014. He turned eighty-six in October 2018.

F. John Lewis

Floyd John Lewis was the closest friend of C. Walton Lillehei. After World War II they worked together at the University of Minnesota under Owen Wangensteen. On September 2, 1952, he performed the first direct-vision open-heart surgery, using hypothermia to preserve the brain function of his five-year-old patient, Jacqueline Johnson. In 1956, Lewis moved to Northwestern University, where he became the first full-time member of the faculty of surgery. After being passed over for the chair of surgery position at Northwestern, Lewis departed for Santa Barbara in 1976 and retired from surgery. He died in Santa Barbara on September 20, 1993, aged seventy-seven.

Walt Lillehei

Clarence Walton Lillehei received his premedical and medical training at the University of Minnesota, earning an undergraduate degree in 1939 and his MD in 1942. During World War II, Lillehei served in the Army Medical Corps in Europe, rising to the rank of lieutenant colonel and earning a Bronze Star for meritorious service. In 1945, he returned to the University of Minnesota and completed his residency under the direction of Owen Wangensteen, then chairman of the Department of Surgery. He pioneered the first cardiac surgical procedures and became known as the father of open-heart surgery. When John

Najarian succeeded Wangensteen, Lillehei left to become professor of surgery and chairman of the Department of Surgery at Cornell University Medical Center and surgeon in chief at New York Hospital. There he undertook a series of multiorgan transplants, including the second clinical transplant of a heart and both lungs in 1969. He died on July 5, 1999, in Minneapolis, of prostate cancer, aged eighty.

Richard Lower

Richard Rowland Lower attended Amherst College and received his medical degree from Cornell University in 1955. While at Stanford he worked with Norman Shumway to develop many of the early experimental techniques for heart transplantation. He subsequently left Stanford to head the cardiac program at the Medical College of Virginia. Lower retired in 1989 to Montana, where he raised cattle. He died of pancreatic cancer on May 17, 2008, aged seventy-eight.

Abdool "Babs" Moossa

Babs Moossa completed his medical school and residency training with honors at the University of Liverpool and United Liverpool Hospitals. In 1972, he was awarded a fellowship in surgery at the Johns Hopkins Hospital and later was recruited to join the faculty at the University of Chicago. In Chicago, he rose quickly to the positions of professor of surgery, vice chairman of the Department of Surgery, chief of the general surgical service and director of surgical research. Moossa then became chairman of surgery at the University of California, San Diego, a post in which he served for twenty-five years. He died on July 17, 2013, from liver cancer, likely a complication from a viral infection sustained after inadvertently pricking his finger during surgery on a patient with hepatitis. He was seventy-three.

John Najarian

John Najarian graduated from the University of California, San Francisco, with a medical degree in 1952 and did his surgical residency there. He then had fellowships at the University of Pittsburg and the Scripps Clinic and Research Foundation in San Diego. He succeeded Owen Wangensteen as the chief of surgery at the University of Minnesota in 1967. For many years he oversaw the sale of a preparation of antilymphocyte serum out of the Department of Surgery, which was illegal under FDA rules. In 1993 he was asked by the university president, Nils Hasselmo, to resign as chairman of the Department of Surgery. In October of that year, the FBI and IRS searched the offices of the Department of Surgery Associates (DSA), Najarian's private practice, seizing his business and financial records, as well as those of DSA's chief financial officer, James Coggins. Coggins was subsequently fired and the process to remove Najarian from his tenured faculty position began. Najarian lost his privileges to conduct research involving human subjects. In February 1995 Najarian resigned from the University Medical School faculty. He was subsequently tried on twenty-two counts of fraud, tax evasion, embezzlement, and other charges. A well-known and locally beloved figure, he was acquitted on all counts that had not already been dismissed by a friendly judge. Najarian lives in Minneapolis. He turned ninety-one in December 2018.

Matt Paneth

Matt Paneth qualified as a doctor at Oxford University, where he worked until he became a resident in surgery at the Brompton Hospital in London. In 1956 he was awarded a Fulbright scholarship and traveled to America to work for a year with Walt Lillehei in Minneapolis. Norman Shumway was a resident there at the same time. After returning to the Brompton, Paneth worked for Lord Brock as senior registrar. Upon

Brock's retirement in 1959, he was appointed to the staff of the Brompton, where he served as consultant surgeon for almost thirty years. When he was ninety-one, a medical examination showed he had lung cancer. He refused treatment and died ten days later, on September 1, 2011.

Ken Porter

Kenneth Porter graduated from St. Mary's Hospital medical school in 1948 and became chair in pathology at St. Mary's in 1967. In the 1950s he worked with Roy Calne, who was studying renal transplantation in dogs. Porter began to document in detail what happened when a kidney transplant was rejected. No one had done this before. Porter later collaborated on the rejection problem with Thomas Starzl, a pioneer in liver transplantation. Porter died on April 13, 2013, aged eighty-eight years.

Norman Shumway

Norman Shumway received his MD from Vanderbilt University in 1949. He did his residency at the University of Minnesota under Walt Lillehei alongside Matt Paneth. Christiaan Barnard was there at the same time. After moving to Stanford University, he pioneered the surgical technique and early management of heart transplantation in the experimental laboratories. On November 20, 1967, he announced that his team was ready to perform a human heart transplant when a suitable donor and patient were found. However, Dr. Christiaan Barnard unexpectedly did the first human heart transplant the next month, in Cape Town, South Africa. Shumway performed the first adult human heart transplant in the US a month later. He went on to make the operation a standard procedure after virtually all other surgeons had abandoned it. He is widely regarded as the father of heart transplantation. He was the first recipient of the Lifetime Achievement Award by the International Society for Heart and Lung Transplantation. He died of cancer on February 10, 2006, in Palo Alto, the day after his eighty-third birthday.

Thomas Starzl

Thomas Earl Starzl attended Northwestern University Medical School in Chicago, where in 1950 he received a master of science degree in anatomy and in 1952 earned both a PhD in neurophysiology and an MD with distinction. He performed the first human liver transplant in 1963 and the first successful human liver transplant in 1967, both at the University of Colorado Health Sciences Center. He subsequently moved to the University of Pittsburgh, where he set up the busiest and most successful transplant institute in the world. He has often been referred to as the father of modern transplantation. Starzl has authored or coauthored more than two thousand scientific articles, three hundred book chapters, and four books. His memoir, *The Puzzle People*, was named by *The Wall Street Journal* as the third best book on doctors' lives. Starzl was presented the National Medal of Science by President George W. Bush at the White House in 2006. In celebration of his eightieth birthday, the University of Pittsburgh renamed one of its newest medical research buildings the Thomas E. Starzl Biomedical Science Tower. Dr. Starzl died on March 4, 2017, aged ninety.

BIBLIOGRAPHY AND SUGGESTED READING

Bannister, Roger. *Twin Tracks*. London: The Robson Press, 2015.

Bonser, Robert S., L S Fragomeni, Jolene M Kriett, M P Kaye and Stuart W. Jamieson. "Technique of clinical double-lung transplantation." The Journal of heart transplantation 7 4 (1988): 298-303.

Greenberg, Mark J., Donald L. Janssen, Stuart W. Jamieson, Abraham Rothman, David D. Frankville, Sheila D. Cooper, Jolene M. Kriett, Pat K. Adsit, Amy L. Shima, Patrick J. Morris, and Meg Sutherland-Smith. "Surgical Repair of an Atrial Septal Defect in a Juvenile Sumatran Orangutan (*Pongo Pygmaeus Sumatraensis*)." *Journal of Zoo and Wildlife Medicine* 30, no. 2 (1999): 256-61. http://www.jstor.org/stable/20095854.

Heaman, E. A. *St. Mary's: The History of a London Teaching Hospital*. London: McGill-Queen's University Press, 2003.

Jamieson, Stuart W., Nelson A. Burton, Charles P. Bieber, Bruce A. Reitz, Philip E. Oyer, Edward B. Stinson, Norman E. Shumway. "Survival of cardiac allografts in rats treated with

Cyclosporin A." *Surgical Forum* 30 (1979): 289–91. https://www.ncbi.nlm.nih.gov/pubmed/395684

Jamieson, Stuart W., Nelson A. Burton, Charles P. Bieber, Bruce A. Reitz, Philip E. Oyer, Edward B. Stinson, Norman E. Shumway. "Cardiac allograft survival in primates treated with Cyclosporin A." *Lancet* 313, no. 8115 (1979): 545. doi: 10.1016/S0140-6736(79)90959-0

Jamieson Stuart W., Vicent Gaudiani, Bruce A. Reitz, Philip E. Oyer, Edward B. Stinson, Norman E. Shumway. "Operative treatment of an unresectable tumor of the left ventricle." *The Journal of Thoracic and Cardiovascular Surgery* 81 (1981): 797–9. https://www.ncbi.nlm.nih.gov/pubmed/6261046

Jamieson, Stuart W., Edward B. Stinson, Phillip E Oyer, J. C. Baldwin and Norman E. Shumway. "Operative technique for heart-lung transplantation." The Journal of thoracic and cardiovascular surgery 87 6 (1984): 930-5.

Jamieson, Stuart, David P. Kapelanski, Naohide Sakakibara, Gerard Manecke, Patricia Thistlethwaite, Kim Kerr, Richard N. Channick, Peter Fedullo, William R Auger. "Pulmonary endarterectomy: experience and lessons learned in 1,500 cases." *The Annals of Thoracic Surgery* 76 (2003): 1457-62. doi:10.1016/S0003-4975(03)00828-2.

Jamieson, Stuart W., Edward B. Stinson, and Norman E. Shumway. "Cardiac Transplantation In 150 Patients at Stanford University." *The British Medical Journal* 1, no. 6156 (1979): 93-95. http://www.jstor.org/stable/25430655.

Miller, G. Wayne. *King of Hearts: The True Story of the Maverick Who Pioneered Open Heart Surgery*. New York: Times Books, 2000.

Starzl, Thomas E. *The Puzzle People: Memoirs of a Transplant Surgeon*. Pittsburgh: University of Pittsburgh Press, 1992.

ACKNOWLEDGEMENTS

I am grateful to several friends who reviewed an early version of the manuscript, but especially to William Souder who worked closely with me and made important suggestions.

SHANE COMES HOME

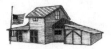

ALSO BY RINKER BUCK

Flight of Passage: A Memoir
First Job: A Memoir of Growing Up at Work

WILLIAM MORROW
An Imprint of HarperCollinsPublishers

SHANE COMES HOME

Rinker Buck

PHOTOGRAPH CREDITS: pages 54, 69, 137, 210: Steven G. Smith/Corbis; 162: Jonna Walker; 238: Steven G. Smith

HarperCollins books may be purchased for educational, business, or sales promotional use. For information please write: Special Markets Department, HarperCollins Publishers Inc., 10 East 53rd Street, New York, NY 10022.

FIRST EDITION

Designed by Renato Stanisic
Illustration of Childers house by Sara Buck

Printed on acid-free paper

Library of Congress Cataloging-in-Publication Data has been applied for.

ISBN 0-06-059325-3

05 06 07 08 09 DIX/RRD 10 9 8 7 6 5 4 3 2 1